Super Chef ABC's

by, Sheri Savory,
Demetra Workman,
and Dakota Workman

Copyright © 2018 by Sheri Savory, Demetra Workman, and Dakota Workman

All rights reserved. No part of this publication may be reproduced, distributed, or transmitted in any form or by any means, including photocopying, recording, or other electronic or mechanical methods, without the prior written permission of the publisher, except in the case of brief quotations embodied in critical reviews and certain other noncommercial uses permitted by copyright law.

ISBN 978-1-7327514-8-4 Paperback http://www.starspublishing.com

Check out Savory's Southern Specialties Cookbook featuring Demetra and Dakota Workman to discover the recipes for many of the items mentioned in this book. Available online at www.walmart.com, www.amazon.com, www.barnesandnoble.com, www.starspublishing.com and many other bookstores around the world.

Thanks, Picmonkey.com for your terrific graphics and to Mrfudge.com for your description of fudge.

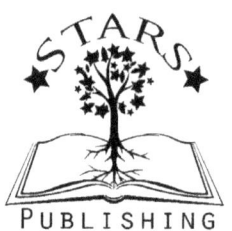

DEDICATED TO SUPER CHEF DEMETRA

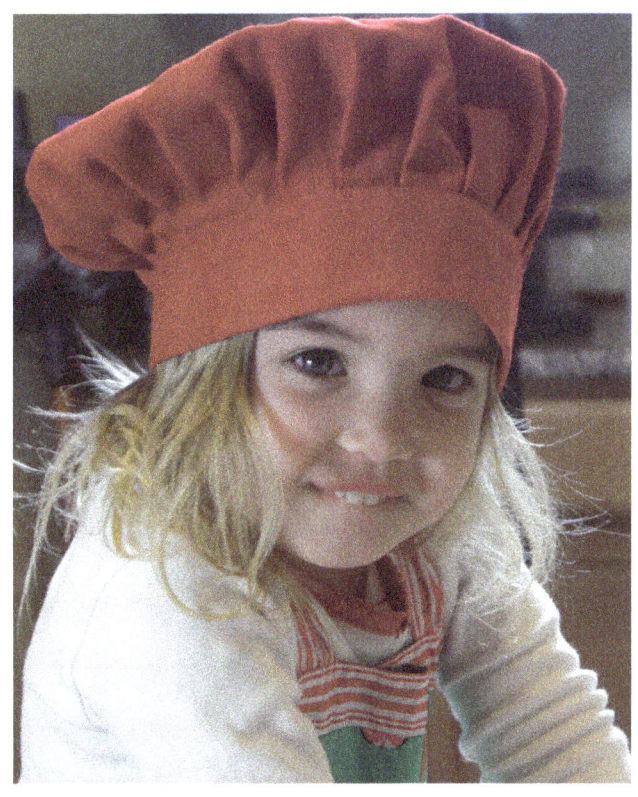

Our special thanks to,
Laure Arnoff, Editor and
Educational Therapist,
Maria Grassu, Pre-K Teacher,
St. Nicholas School,
Rochelle Savory, Supermom,
and Uncle Scott Bailey for
your creative genius and input.

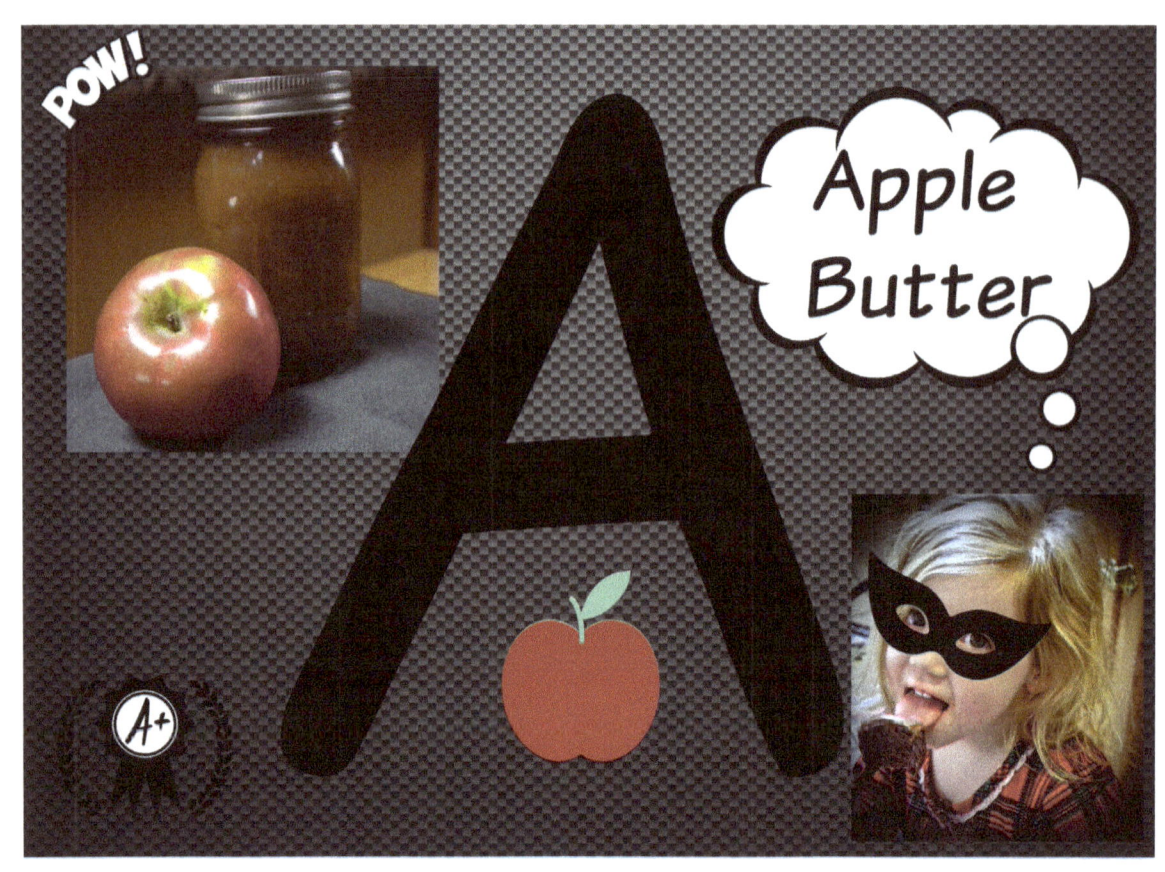

Apple butter tastes great on toast and biscuits.

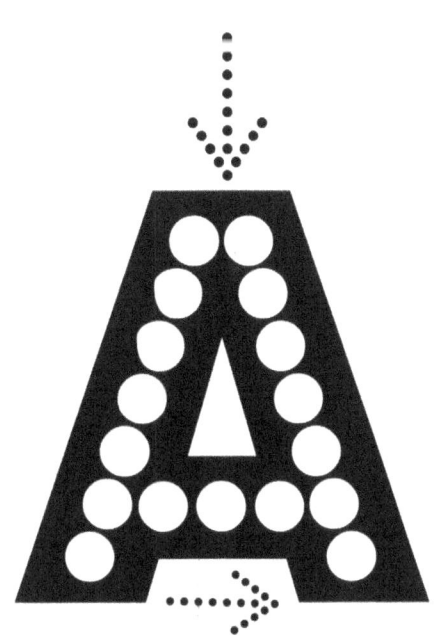

A is for Apple.

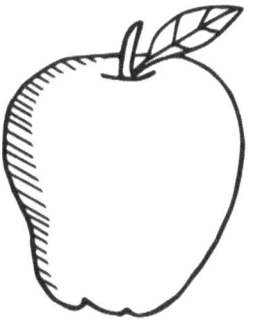

Aa

Practice writing the letter A.

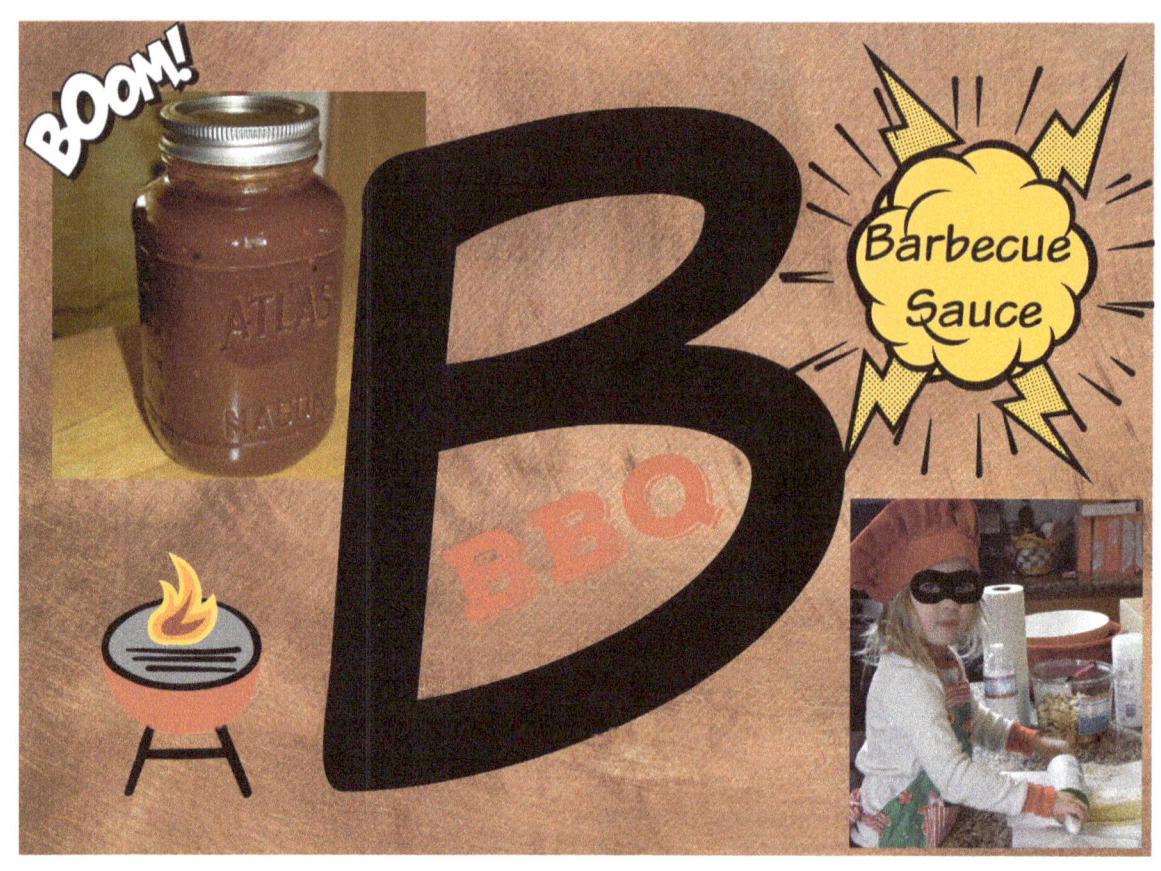

Barbecue sauce is terrific on hamburgers and chicken.

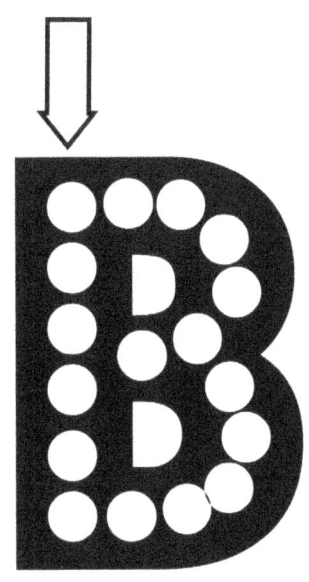

B is for Barbecue.

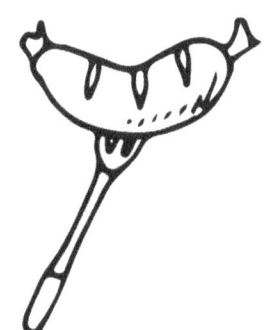

Bb

Practice writing the letter B.

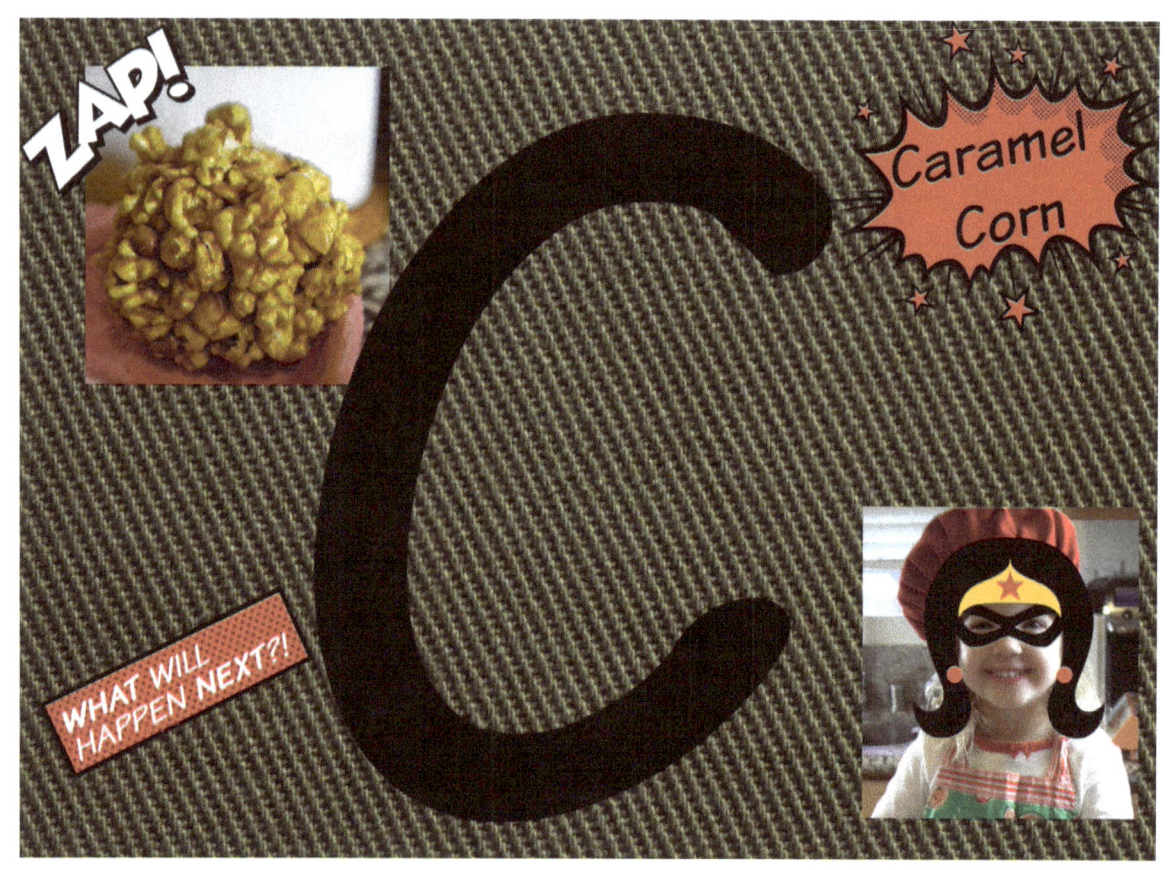

Caramel Corn
is crunchy
and sweet.

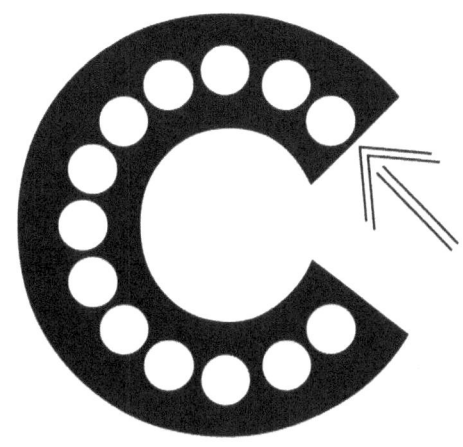

C is for Cookie.

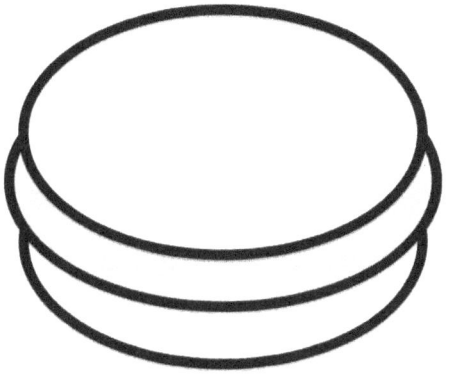

Cc

Practice writing the letter C.

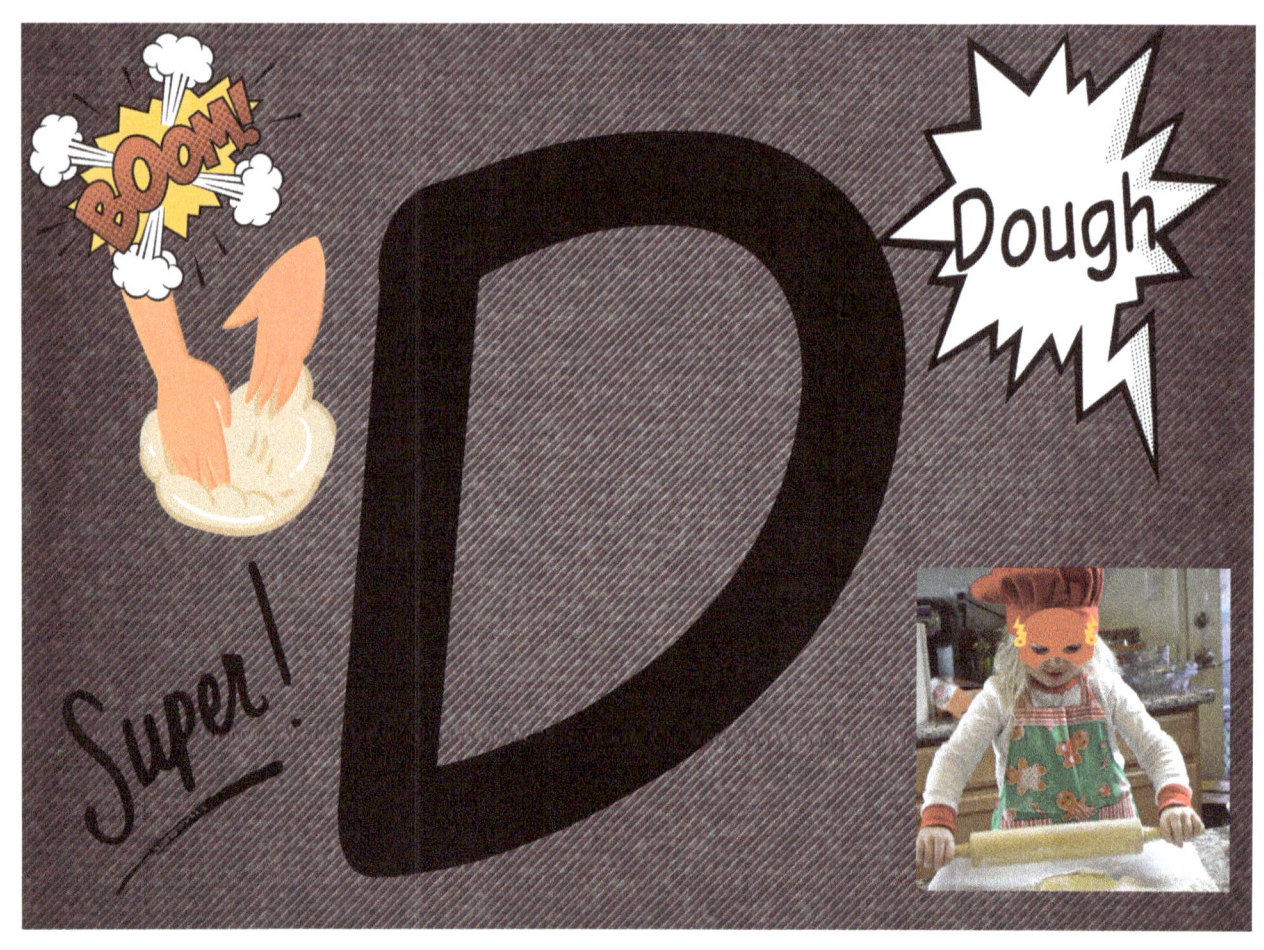

Donut dough comes from ingredients like flour, sugar, and yeast.

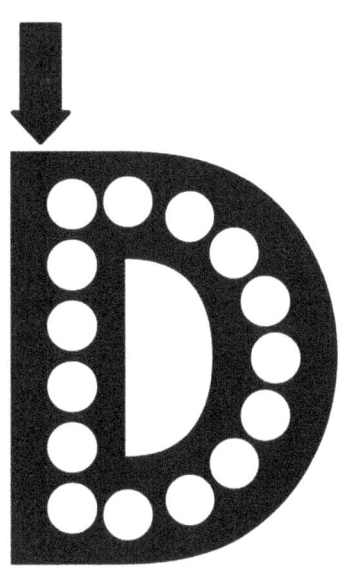

D is for Donut.

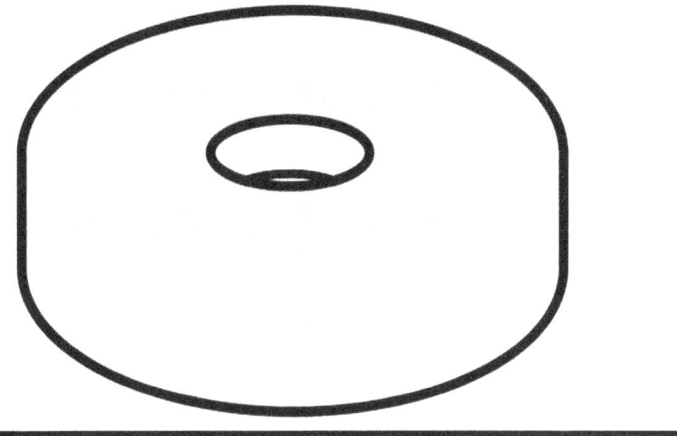

Dd

Practice writing the letter D.

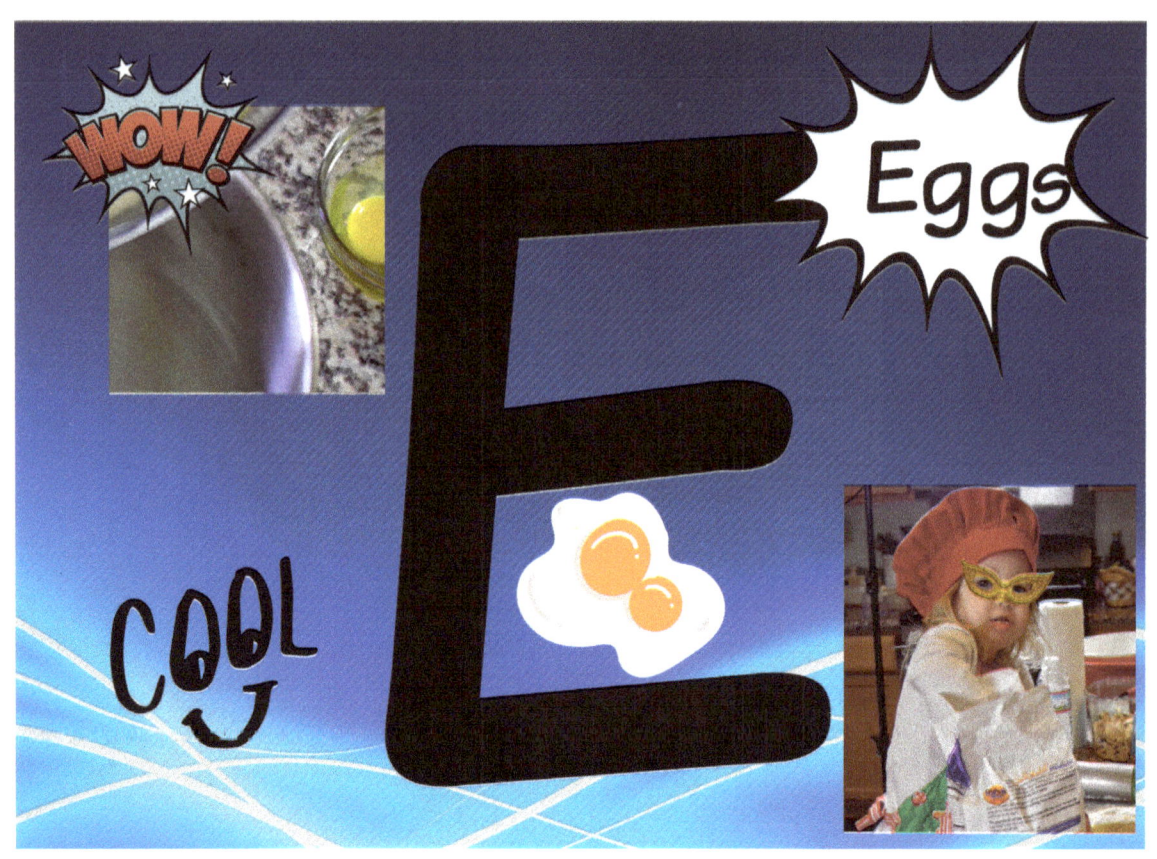

Eggs make baked goods rise so they can be fluffy.

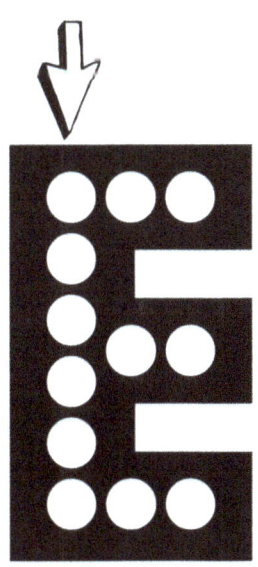

E is for Egg.

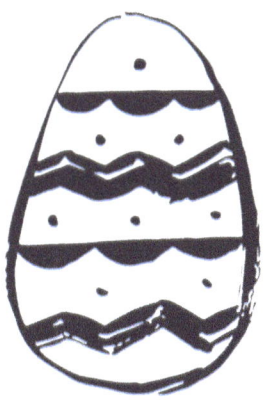

Ee

Practice writing the letter E.

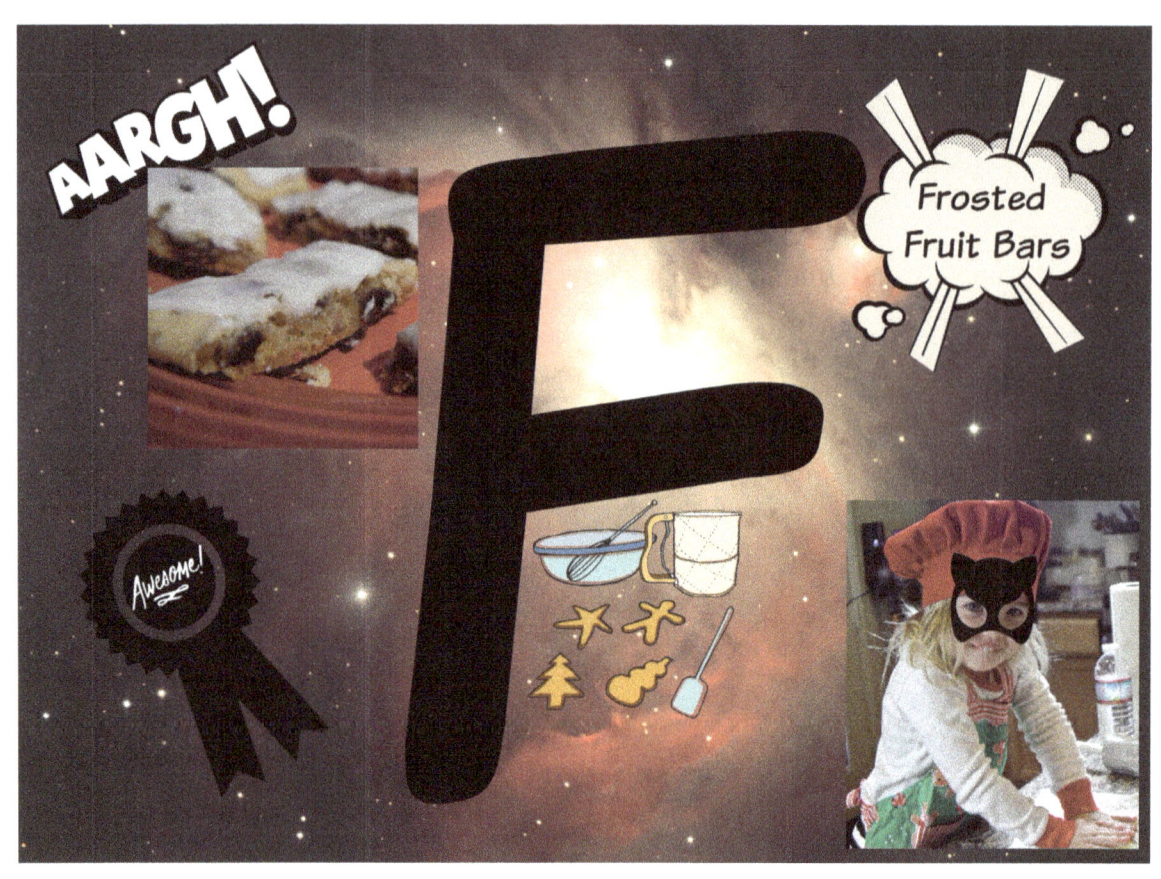

Frosted Fruit Bars are chewy with raisins and candied fruit.

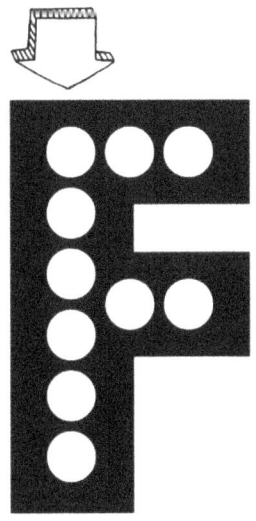

F is for Fruit.

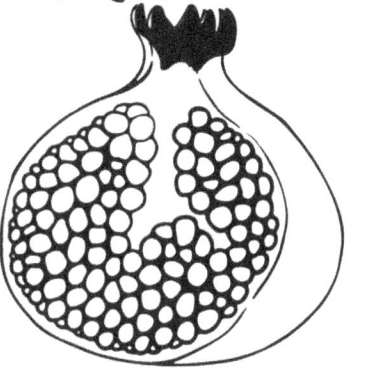

POMEGRANATE

Ff

Practice writing the letter F.

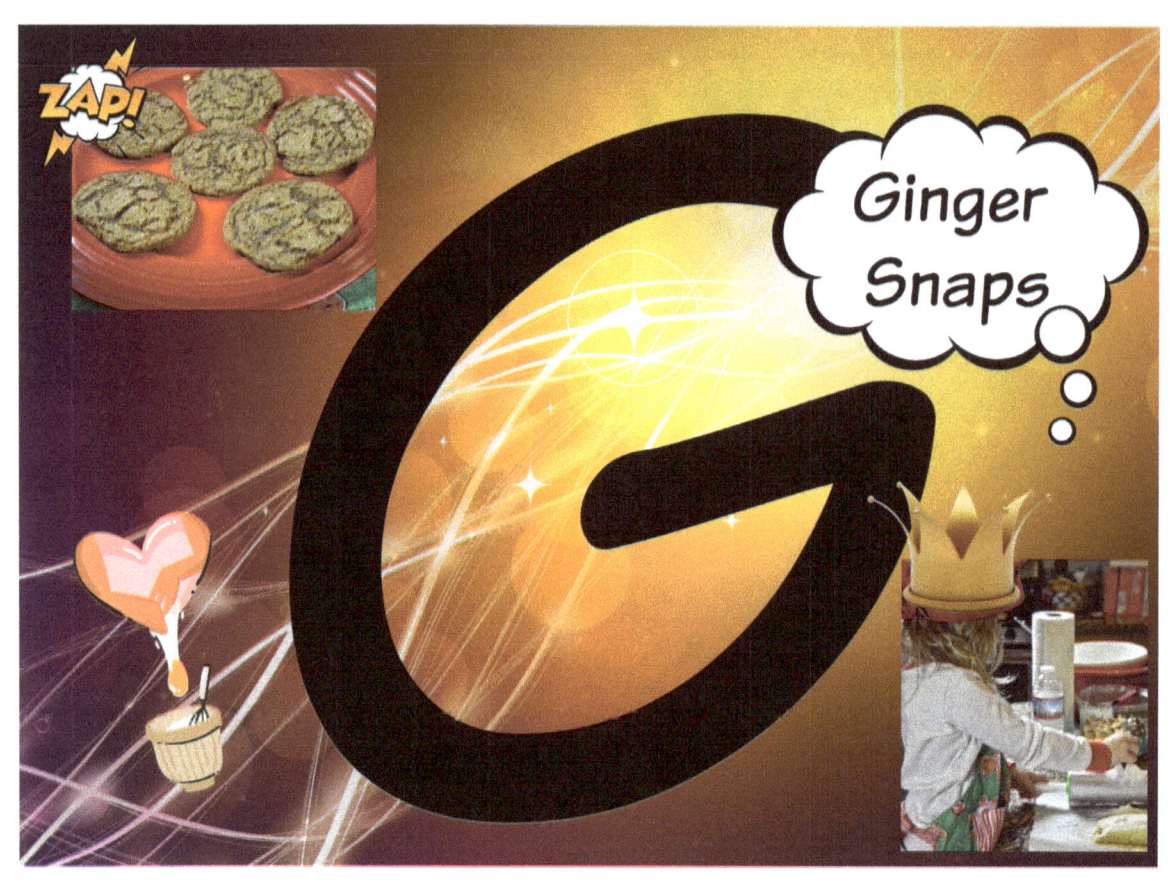

Ginger is a spice from China that gives food a unique flavor.

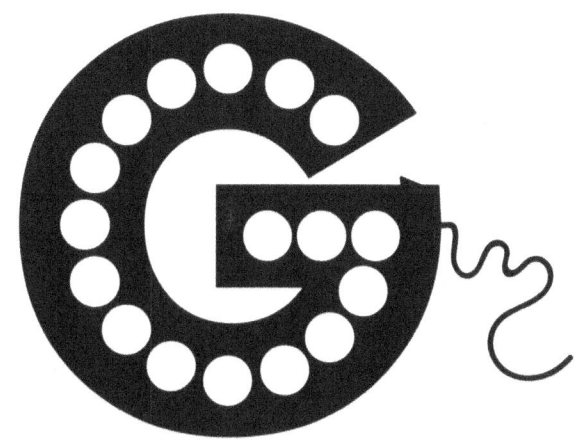

G is for Ginger.

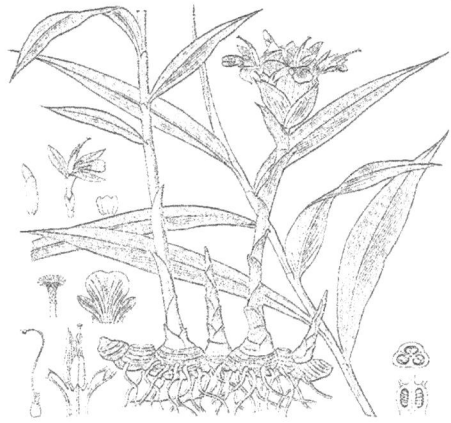

GINGER IS A SPICE THAT ADDS FLAVOR.

Gg

Practice writing the letter G.

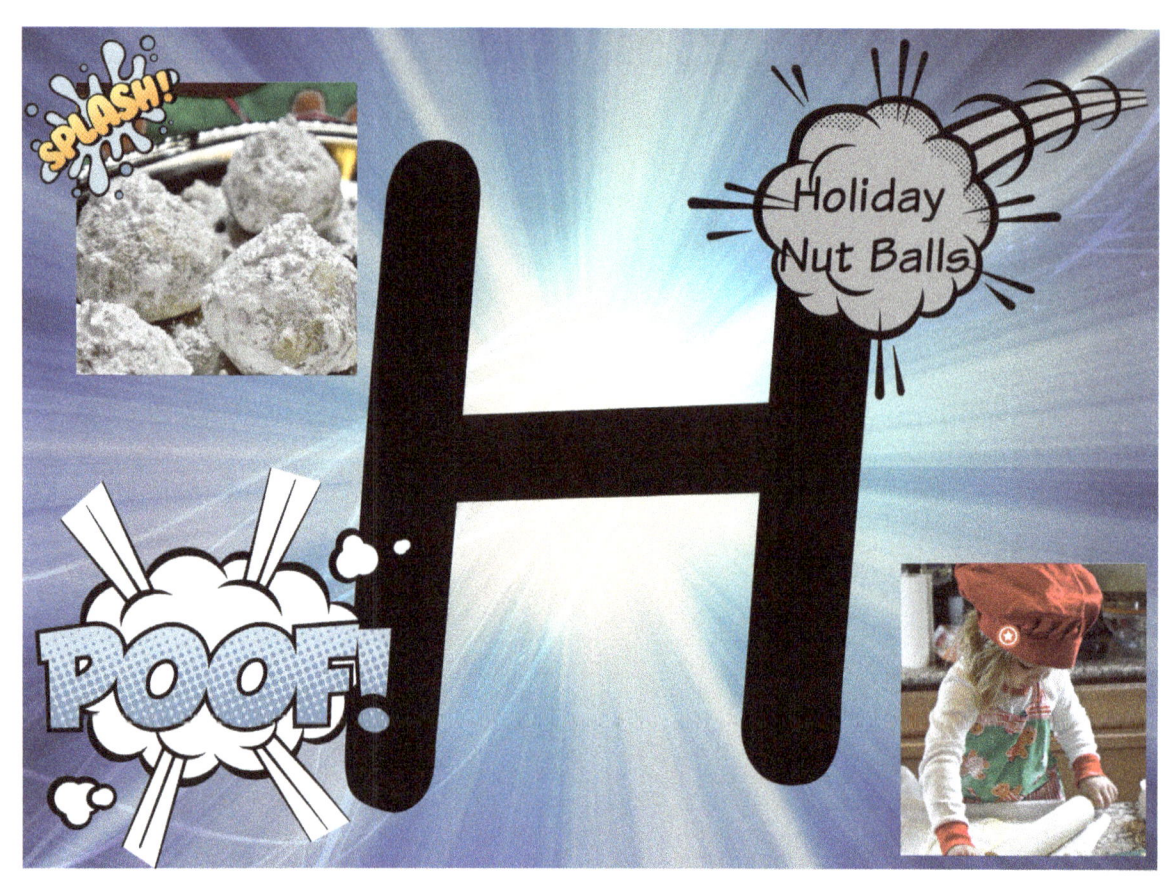

Holiday Nutballs
are buttery,
crunchy and rolled
in powdered sugar.

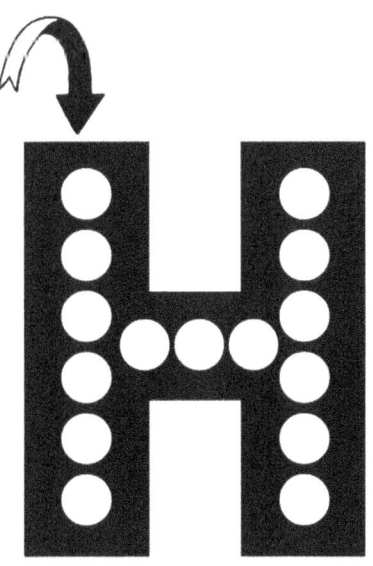

H is for Hamburger.

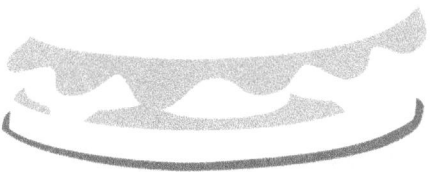

HAMBURGERS ARE MADE FROM MEAT OR VEGGIES.

Hh

Practice writing the letter H.

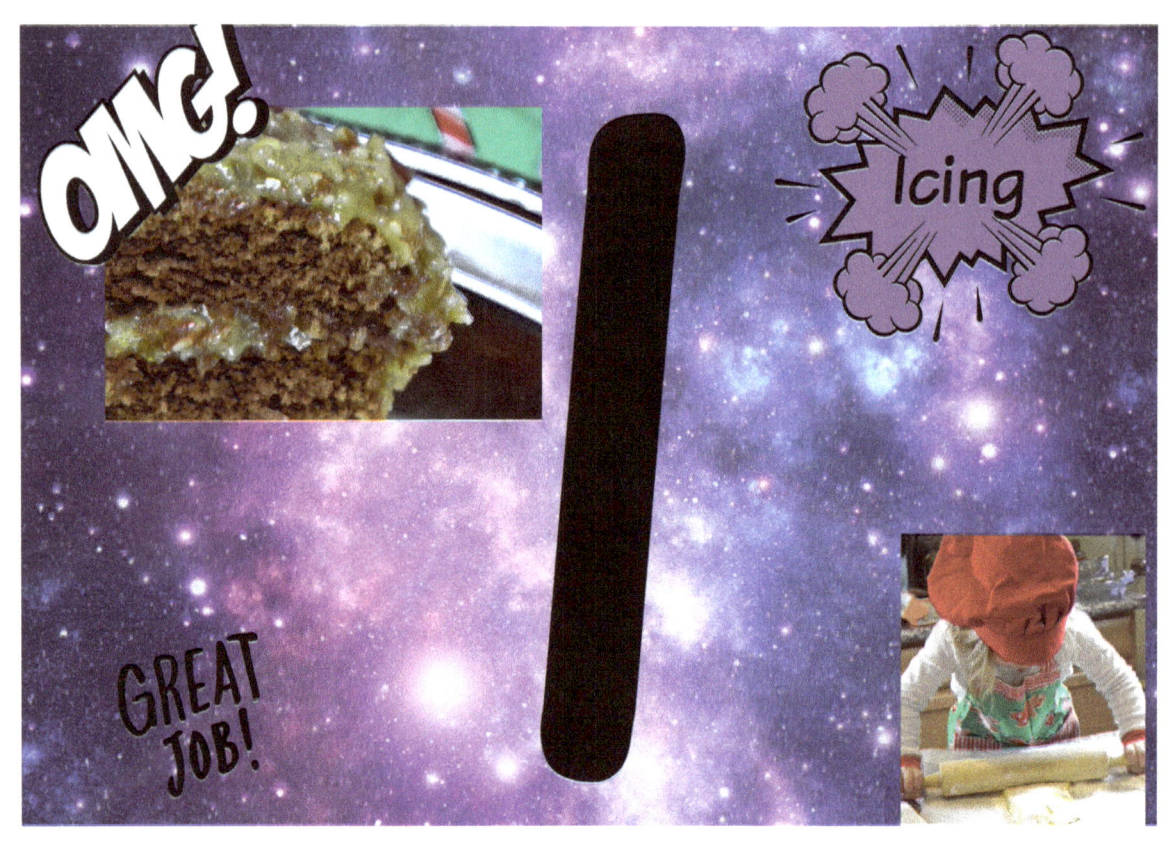

Icing goes on cupcakes and cakes to keep them moist.

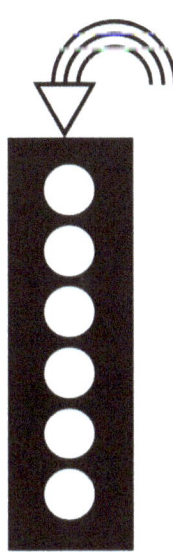

I is for Ice Cream.

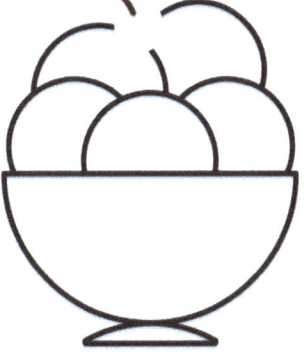

ICE CREAM IS GOOD ON PIE.

Ii

Practice writing the letter I.

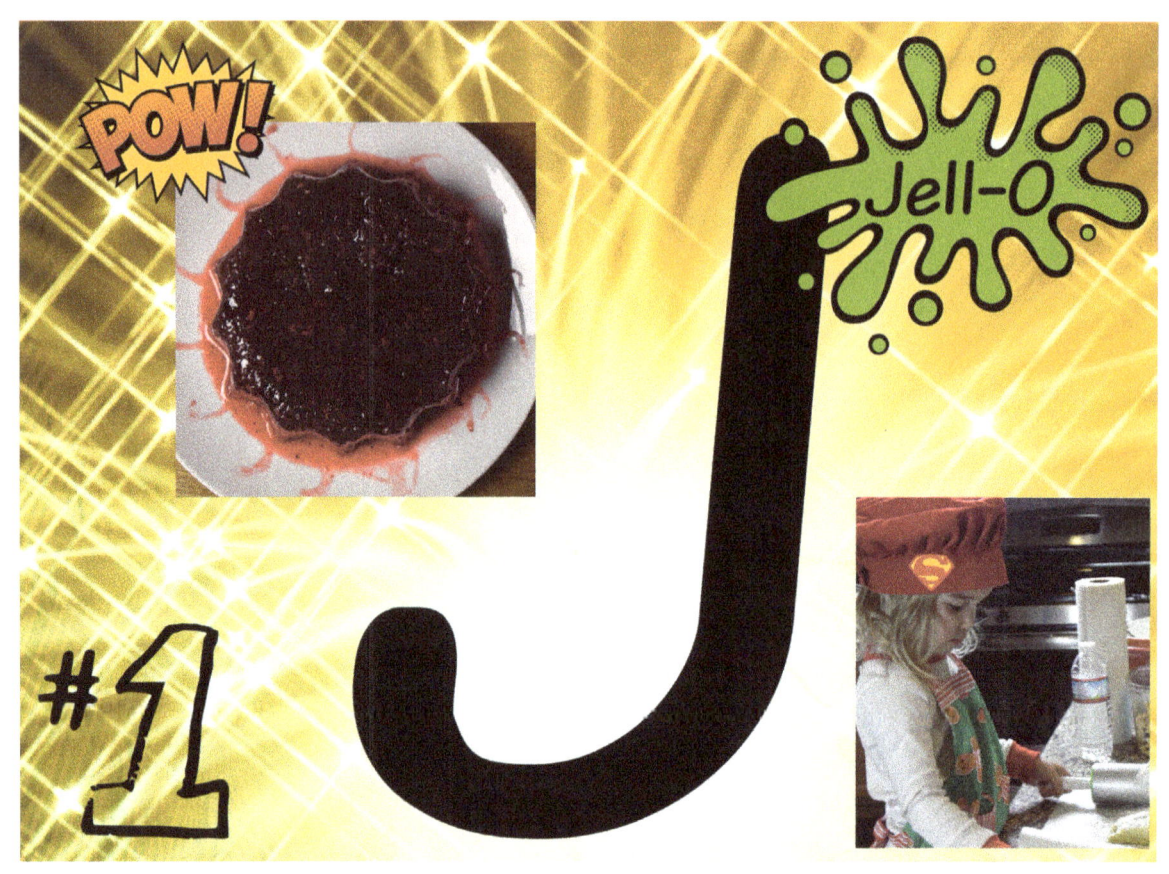

Jell-O Salad is made by mixing fruit and nuts into Jell-O.

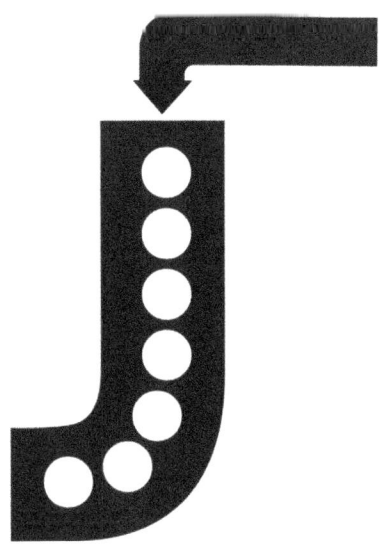

J is for Jelly Beans.

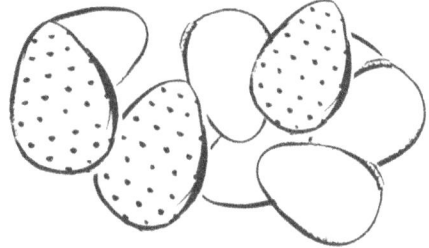

JELLY BEANS ARE MADE IN MANY FLAVORS.

Jj

Practice writing the letter J.

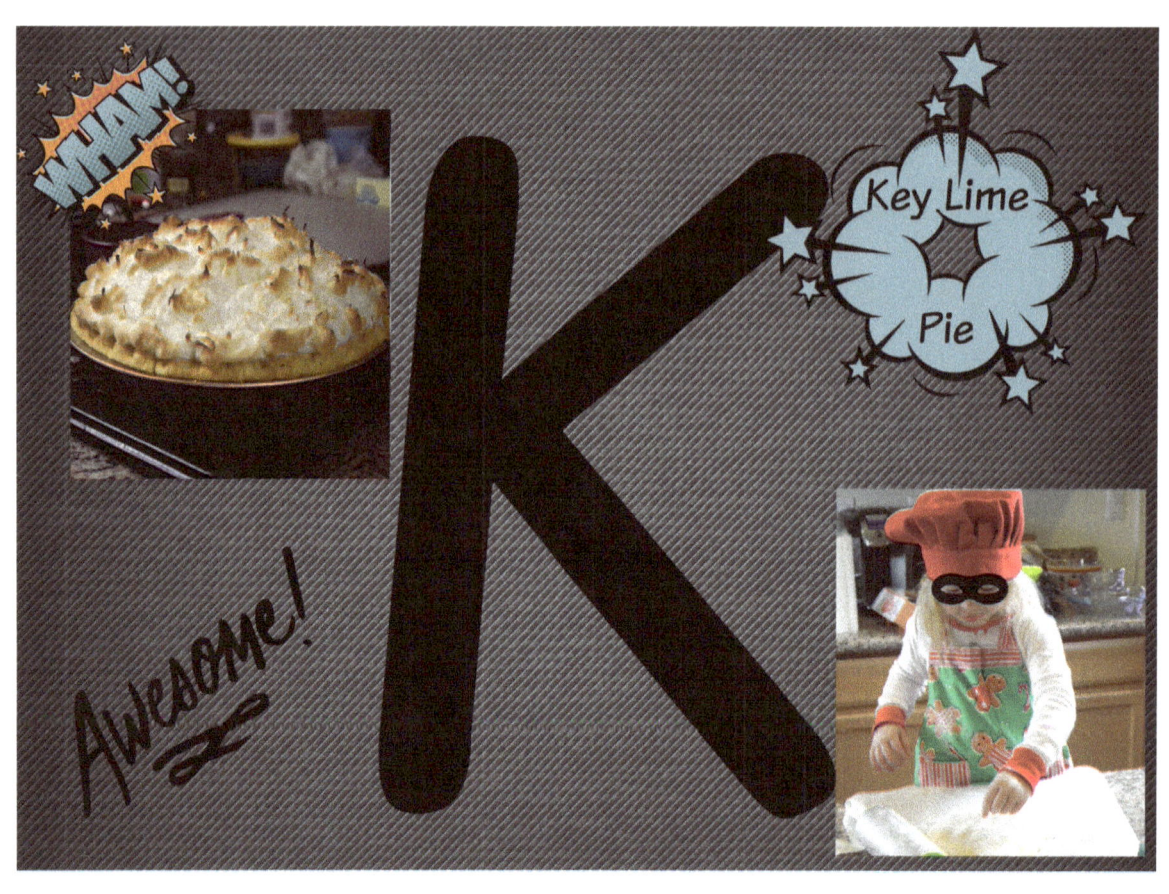

Key Lime Pie begins with a lime called a "Key Lime."

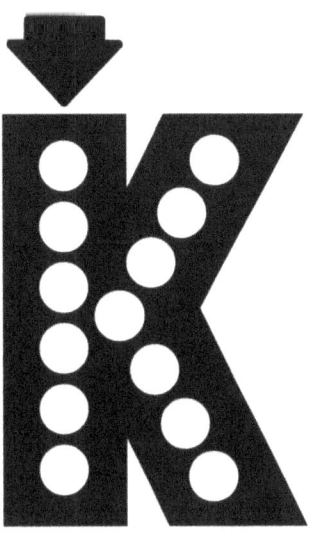

K is for Kabob.

TRY VEGGIES OR MEAT IN YOUR KABOB.

Kk

Practice writing the letter K.

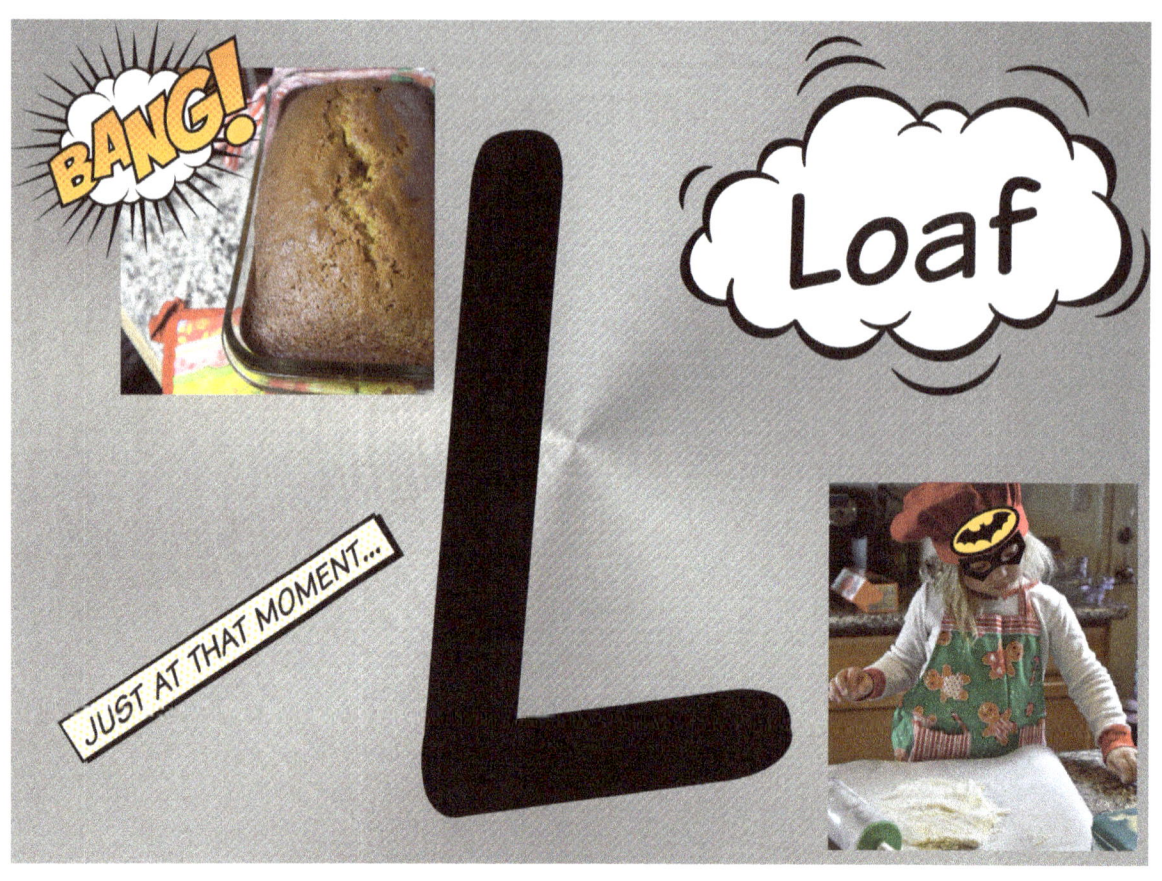

Loaves of bread can be found all around the world.

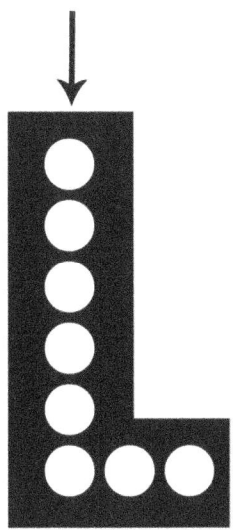

L is for Loaf.

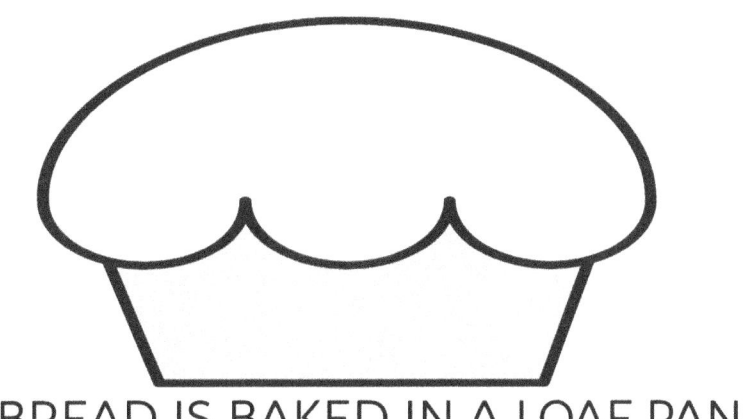

BREAD IS BAKED IN A LOAF PAN.

Practice writing the letter L.

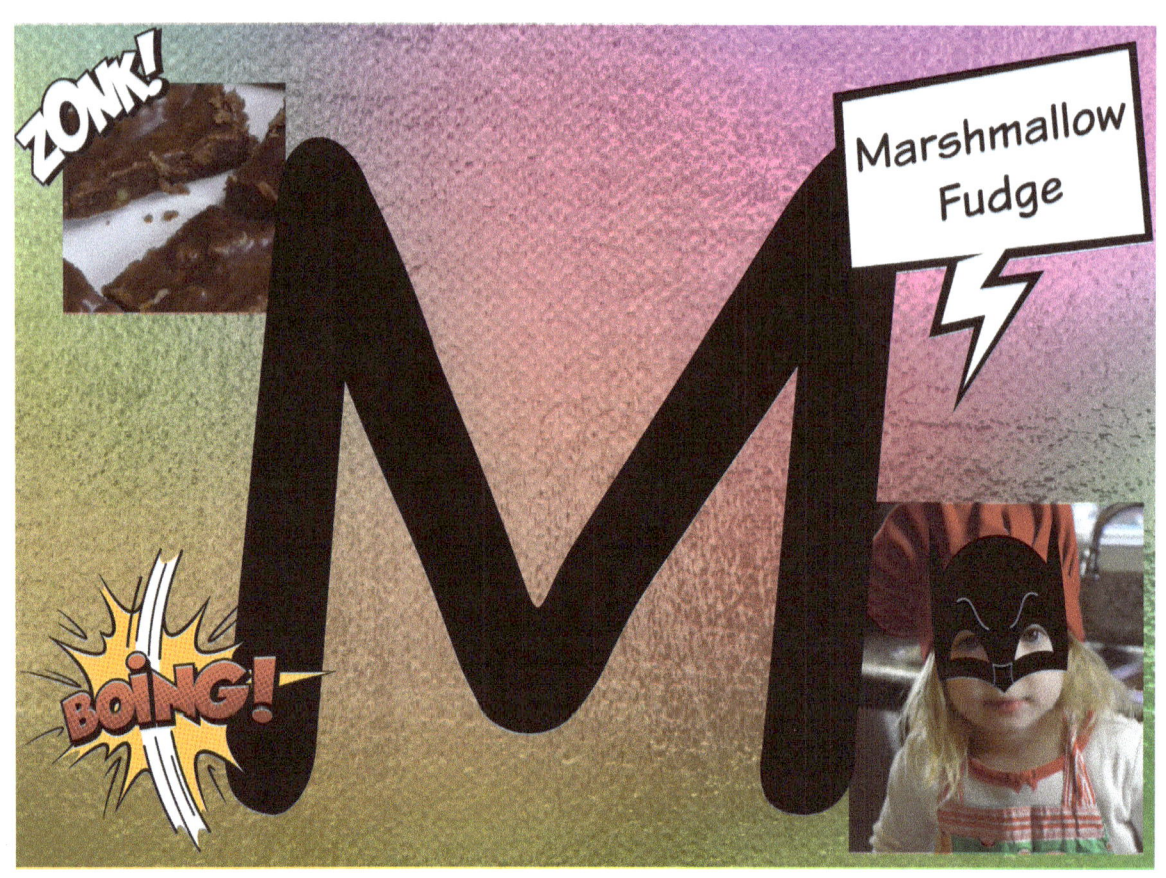

Marshmallow Fudge tastes like a chocolate bar, and a brownie collided.

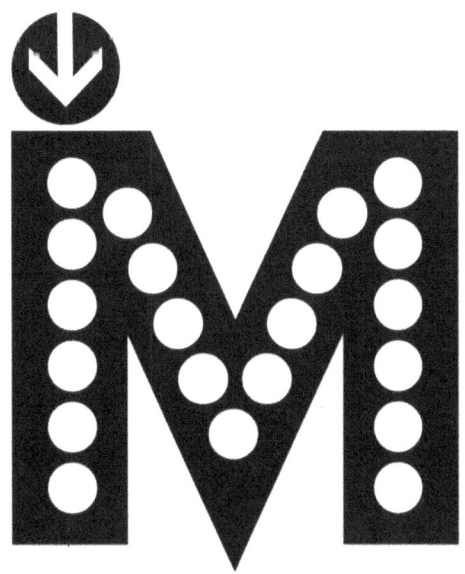

M is for Meat.

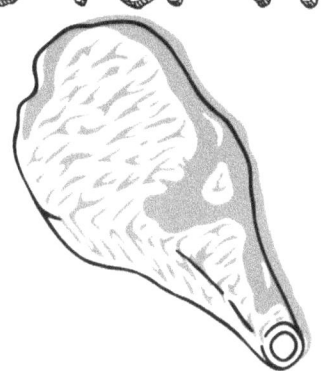

MEAT COMES FROM ANIMALS AND IS HIGH IN PROTIEN.

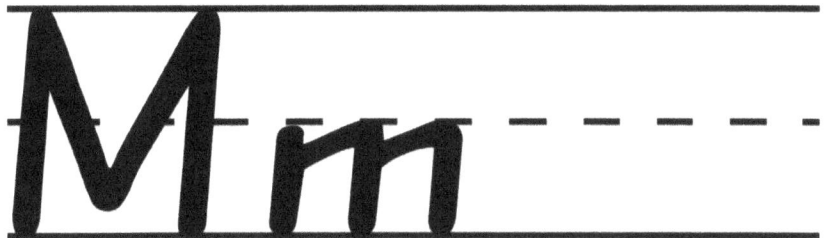

Practice writing the letter M.

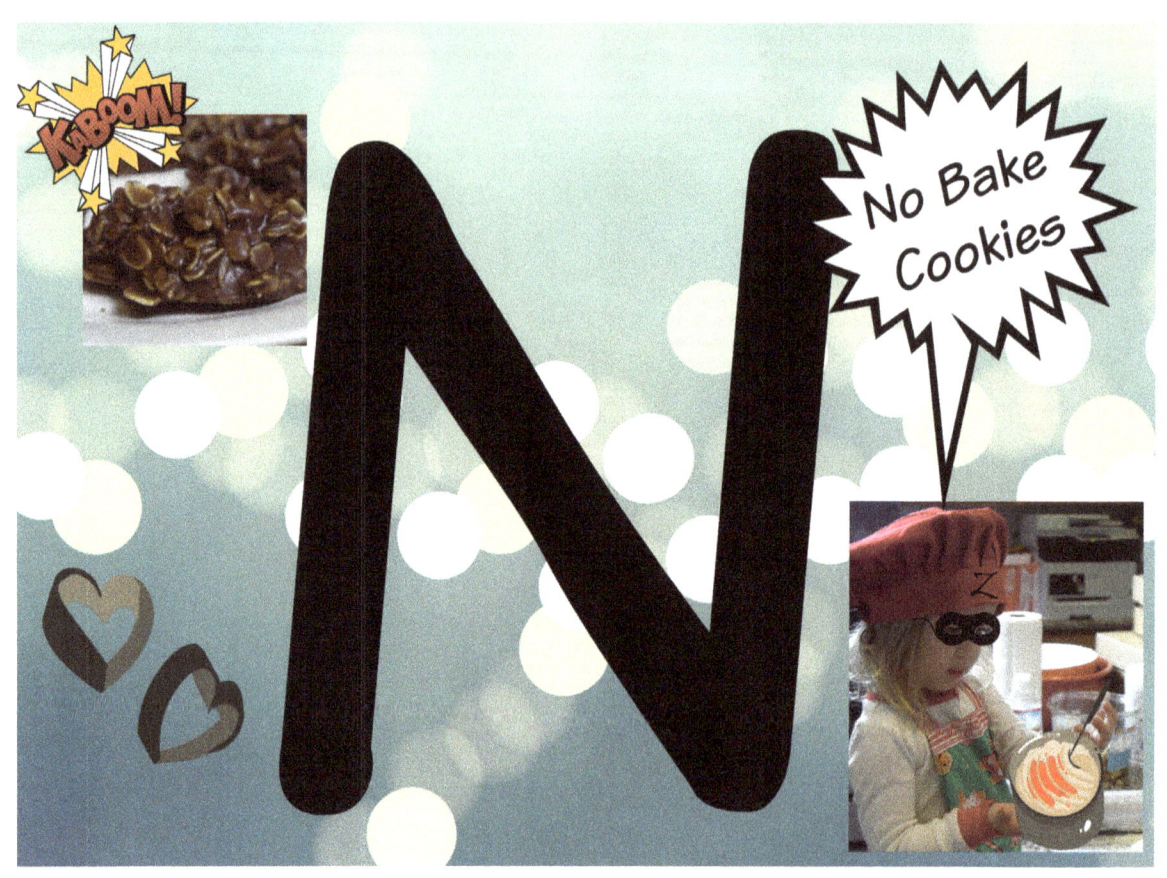

No bake cookies are made from cocoa, oatmeal butter and peanut butter.

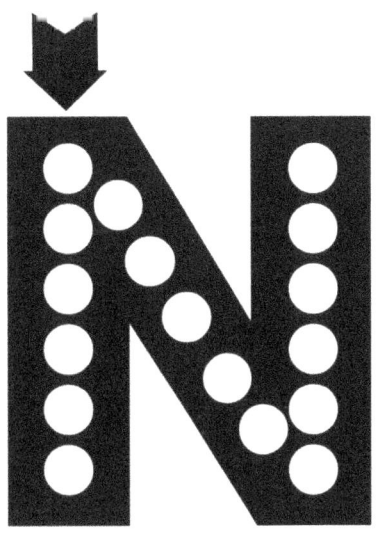

N is for Nectarines.

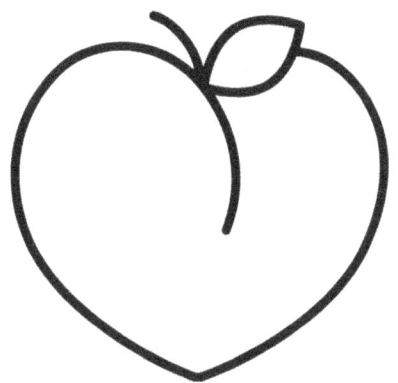

LIKE PEACHES THIS FRUIT IS VERY JUICY.

Nn

Practice writing the letter N.

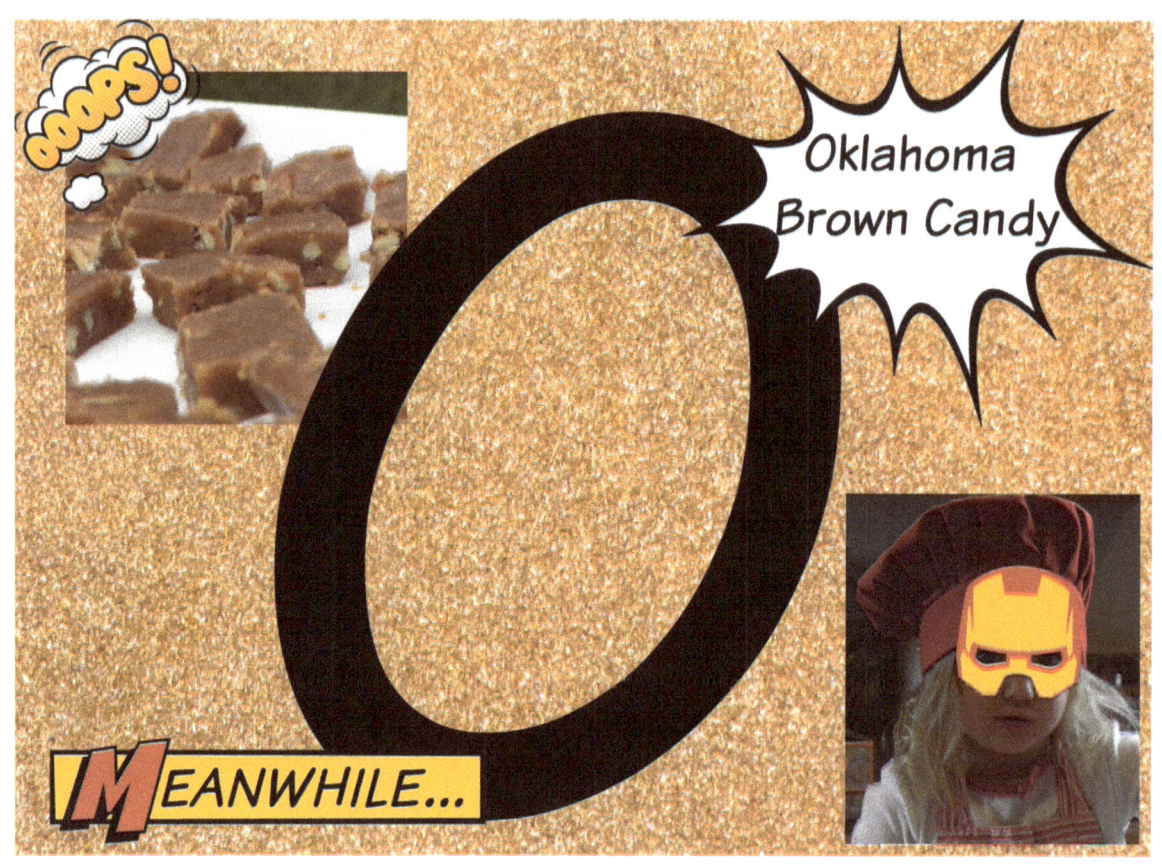

Oklahoma Brown Candy is an unusual brown sugar fudge.

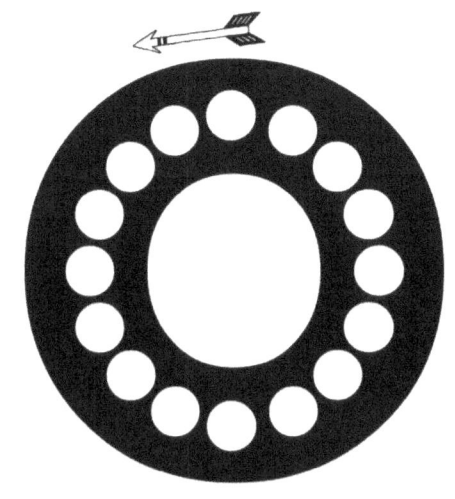

O is for Oil.

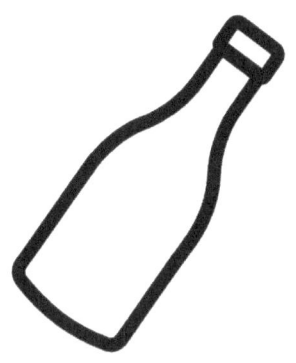

OIL IS USED FOR COOKING AND IN SALADS.

Practice writing the letter O.

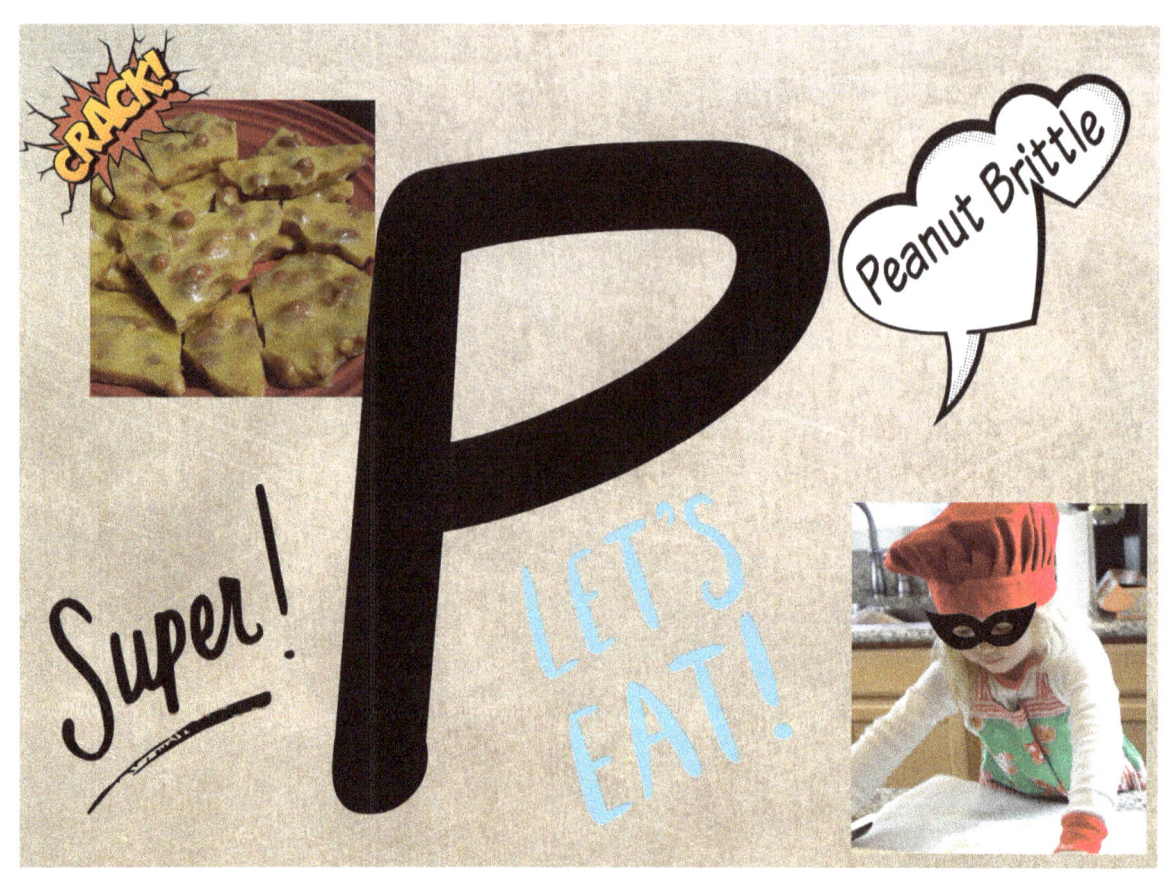

Peanut Brittle is a nutty, buttery candy with a caramel flavor.

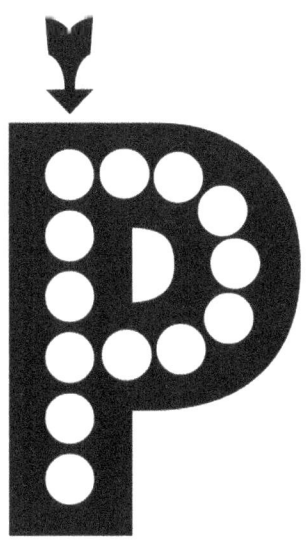

P is for Pizza.

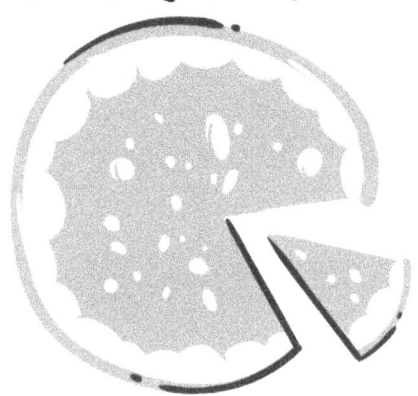

PIZZA IS THE ITALIAN WORD FOR PIE.

Pp

Practice writing the letter P.

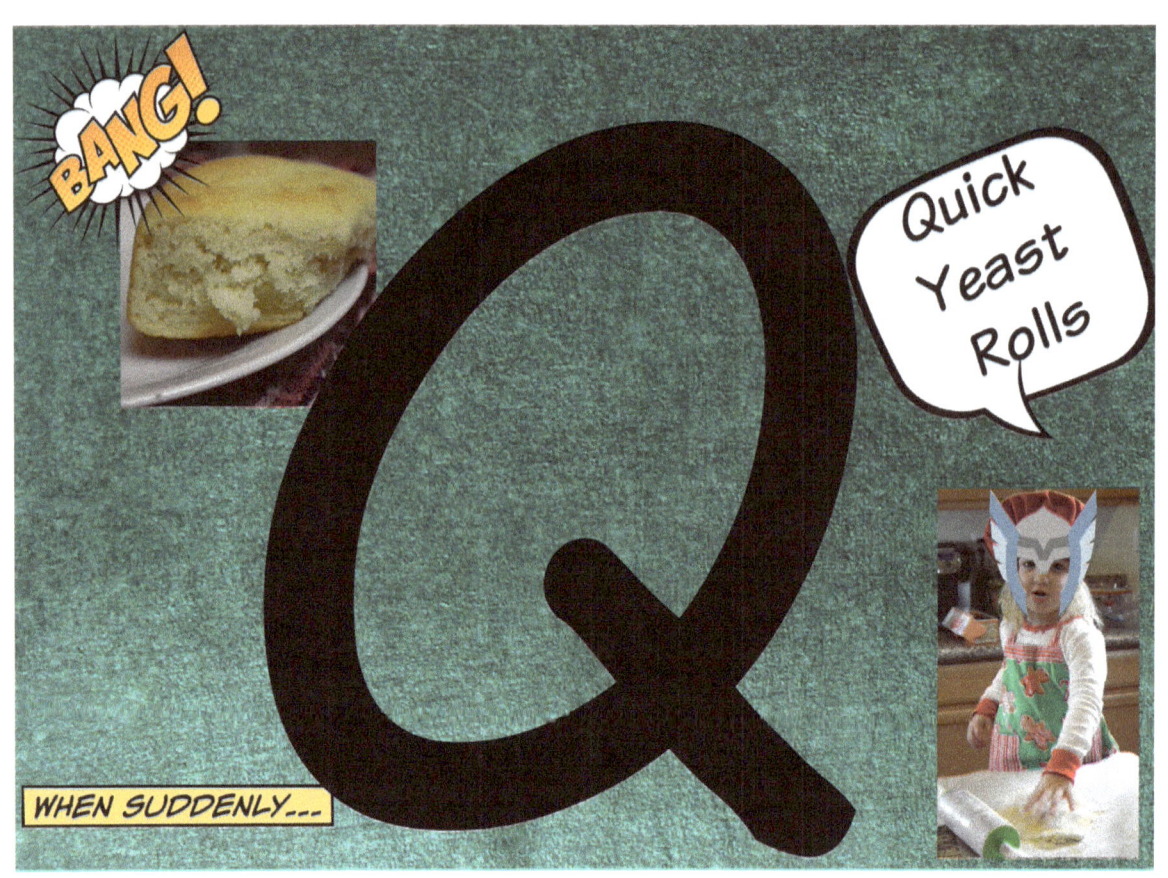

Quick Yeast Rolls are delicious when topped with butter.

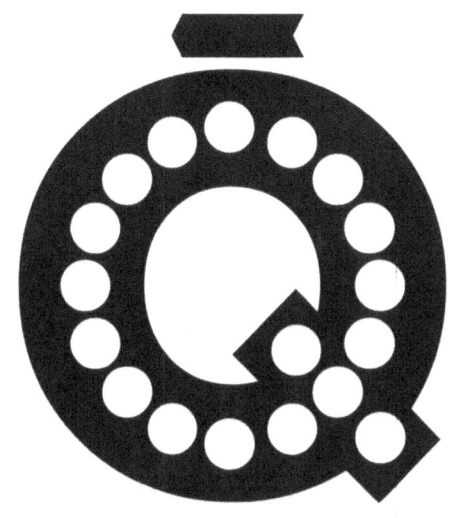

Q is for Quaker oats.

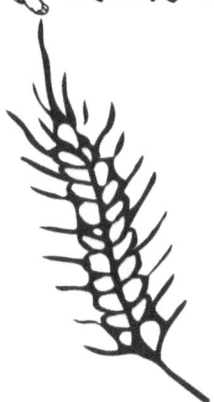

TRY QUAKER OATS IN YOUR NO BAKE COOKIES.

Qq

Practice writing the letter Q.

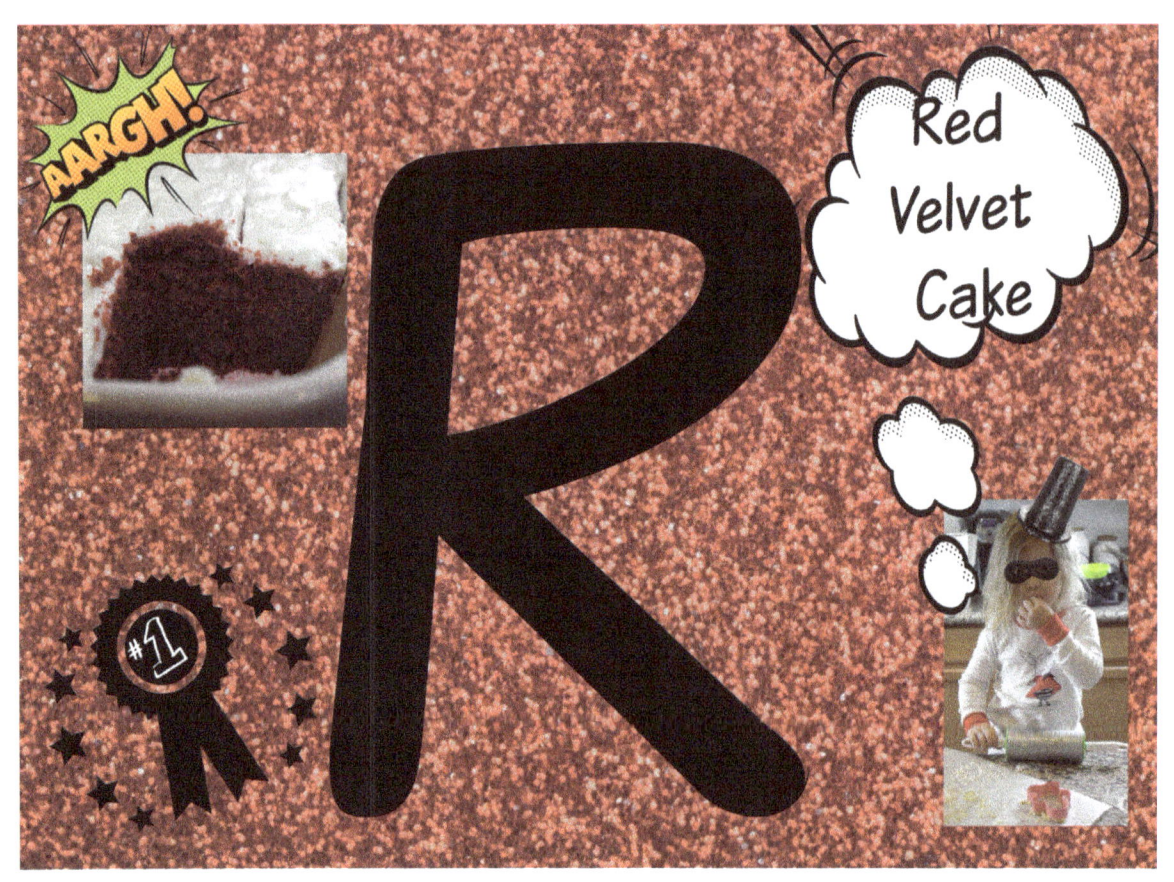

Red Velvet Cake
is a moist,
red-colored,
chocolate cake.

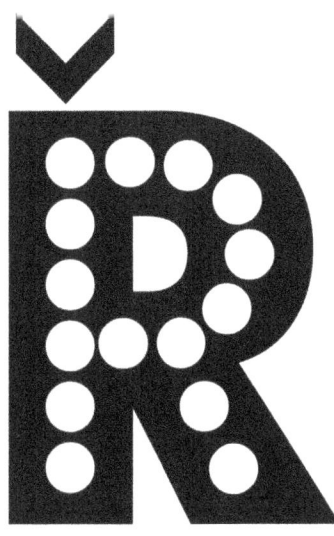

R is for Red Velvet.

RED VELVET CAKE IS A CHOCOLATE CAKE.

Rr

Practice writing the letter R.

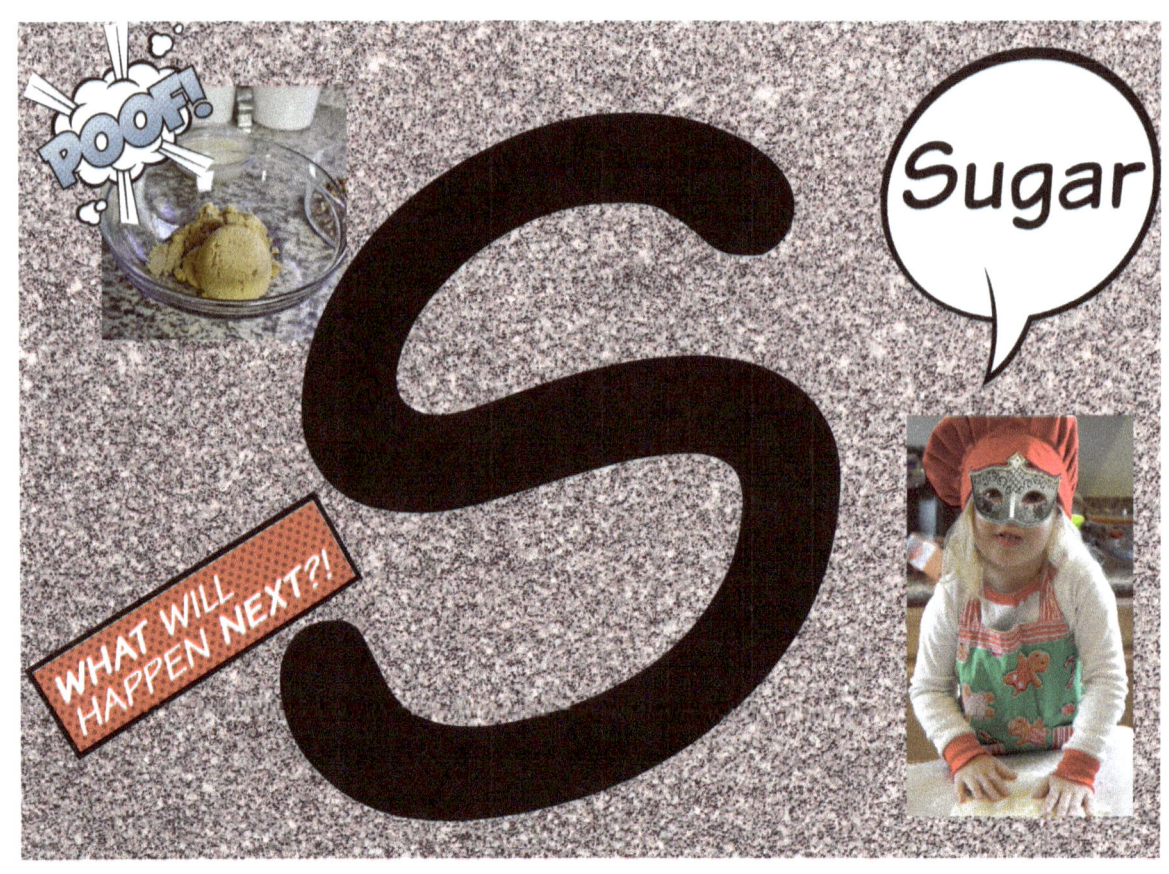

Sugar makes food sweet and is used in cooking.

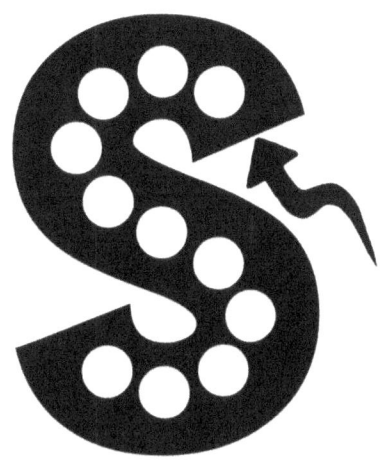

S is for Sugar.

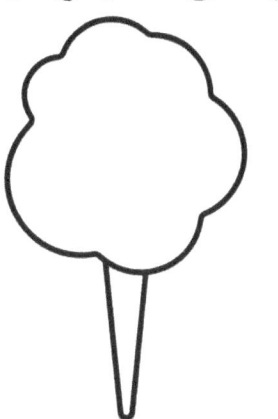

COTTON CANDY IS SIMPLY SPUN SUGAR.

Ss

Practice writing the letter S.

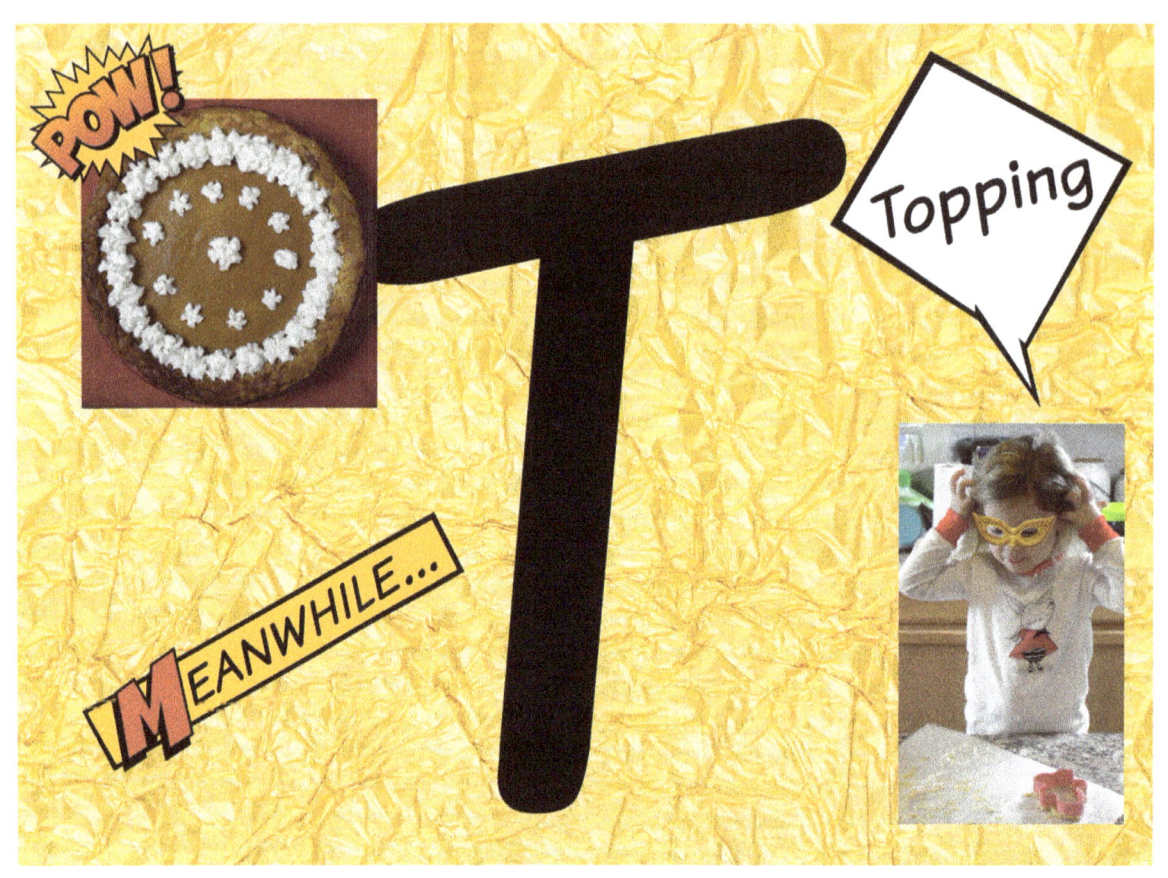

Topping, made from cream is so yummy on Pumpkin Pie.

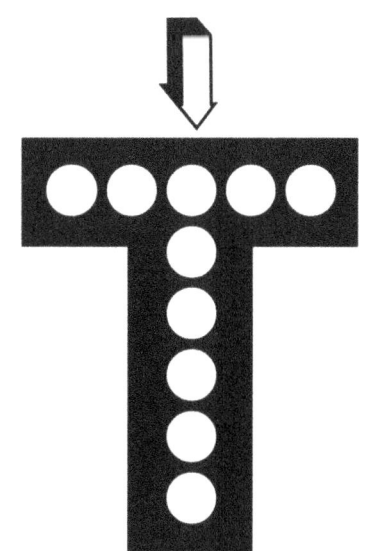

T is for Tuna.

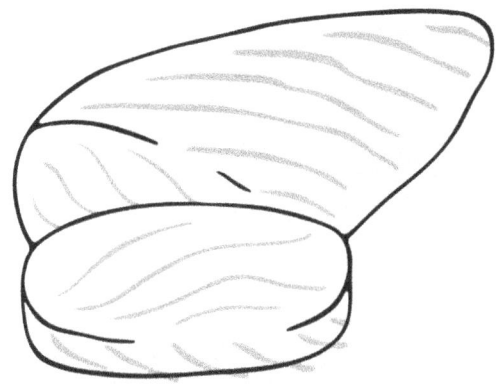

TUNA IS HIGH IN OMEGA 3'S.

Tt

Practice writing the letter T.

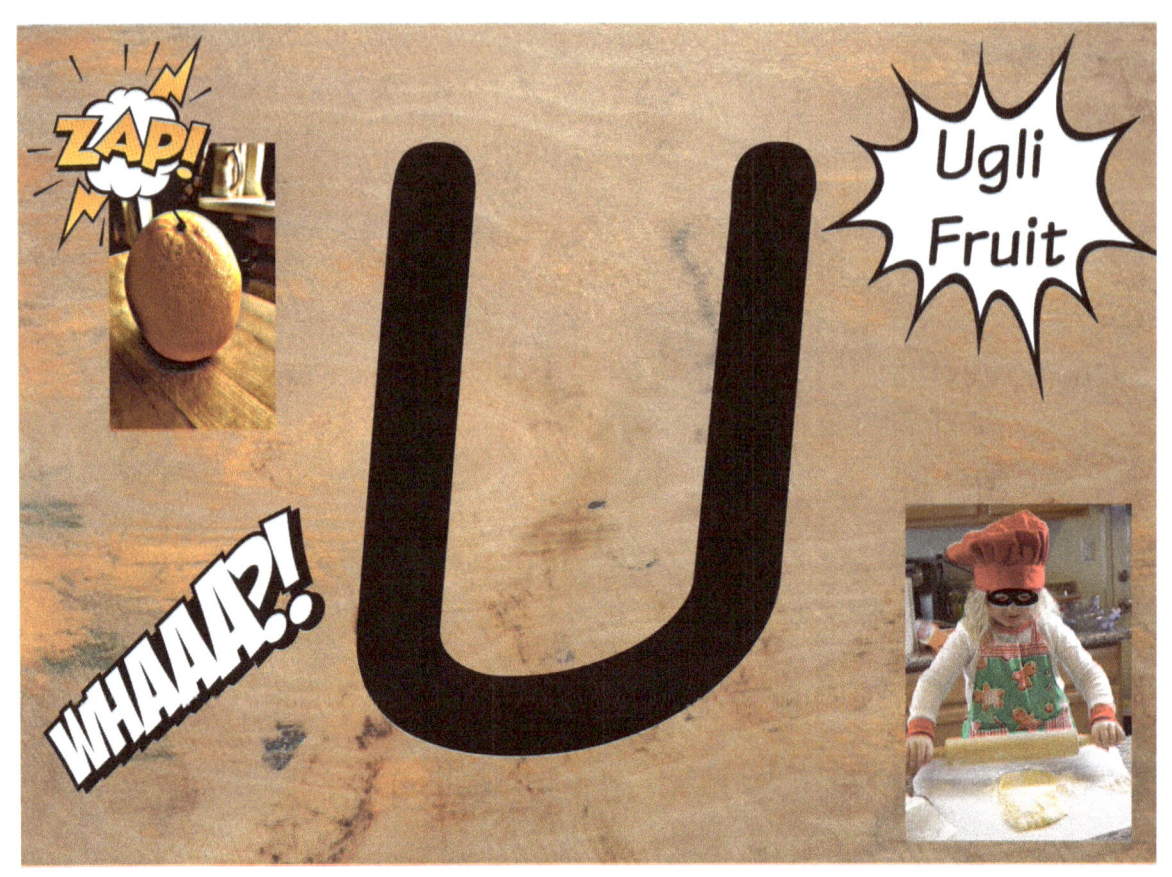

Ugli Fruit is a Jamaican Tangelo.

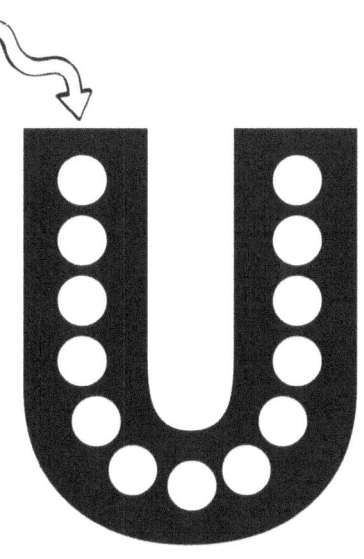

U is for Upside Down Cake.

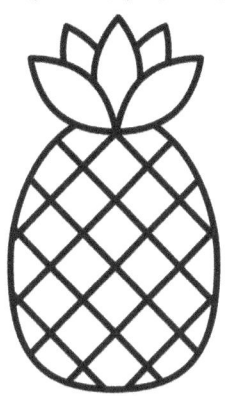

THIS CAKE IS MADE FROM YELLOW CAKE, BROWN SUGAR AND PINEAPPLE.

Uu

Practice writing the letter U.

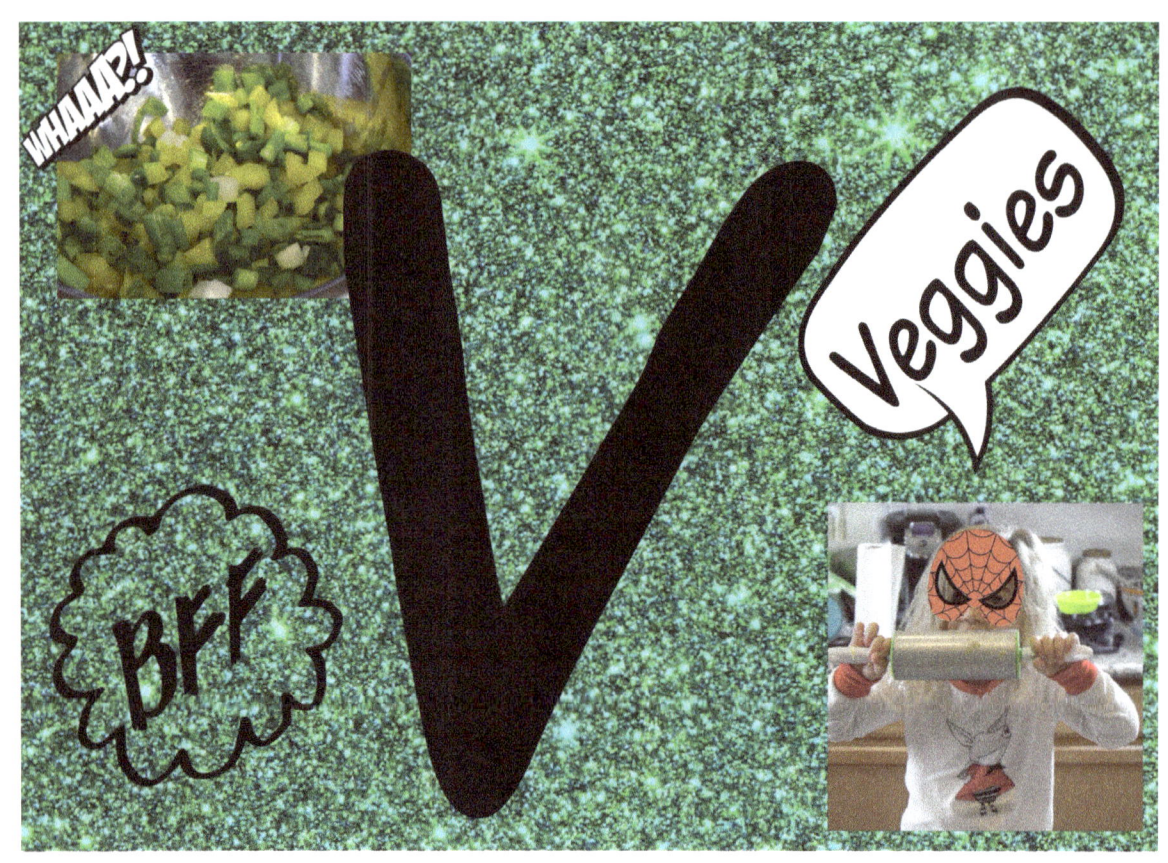

Veggies are a good source of vitamins.

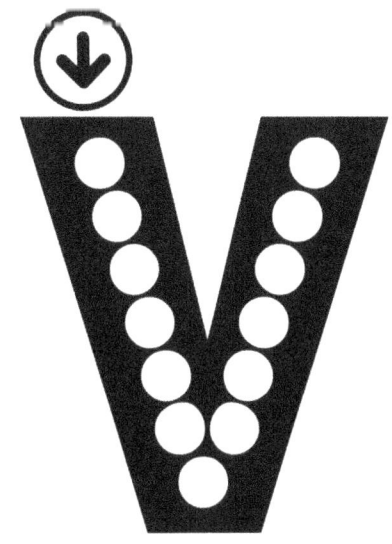

V is for Vegetable Juice.

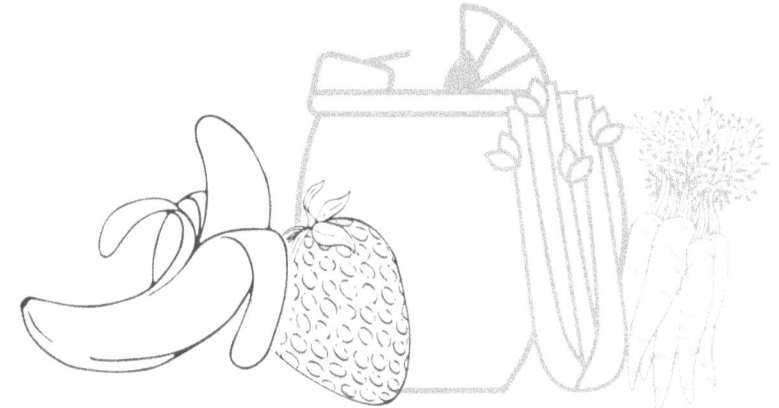

JUICES WITH FRUIT AND VEGGIES TASTE DELICIOUS.

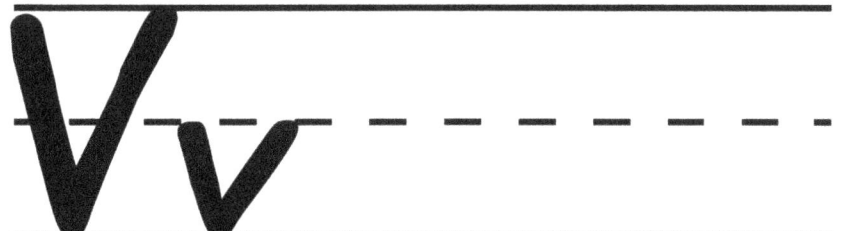

Practice writing the letter V.

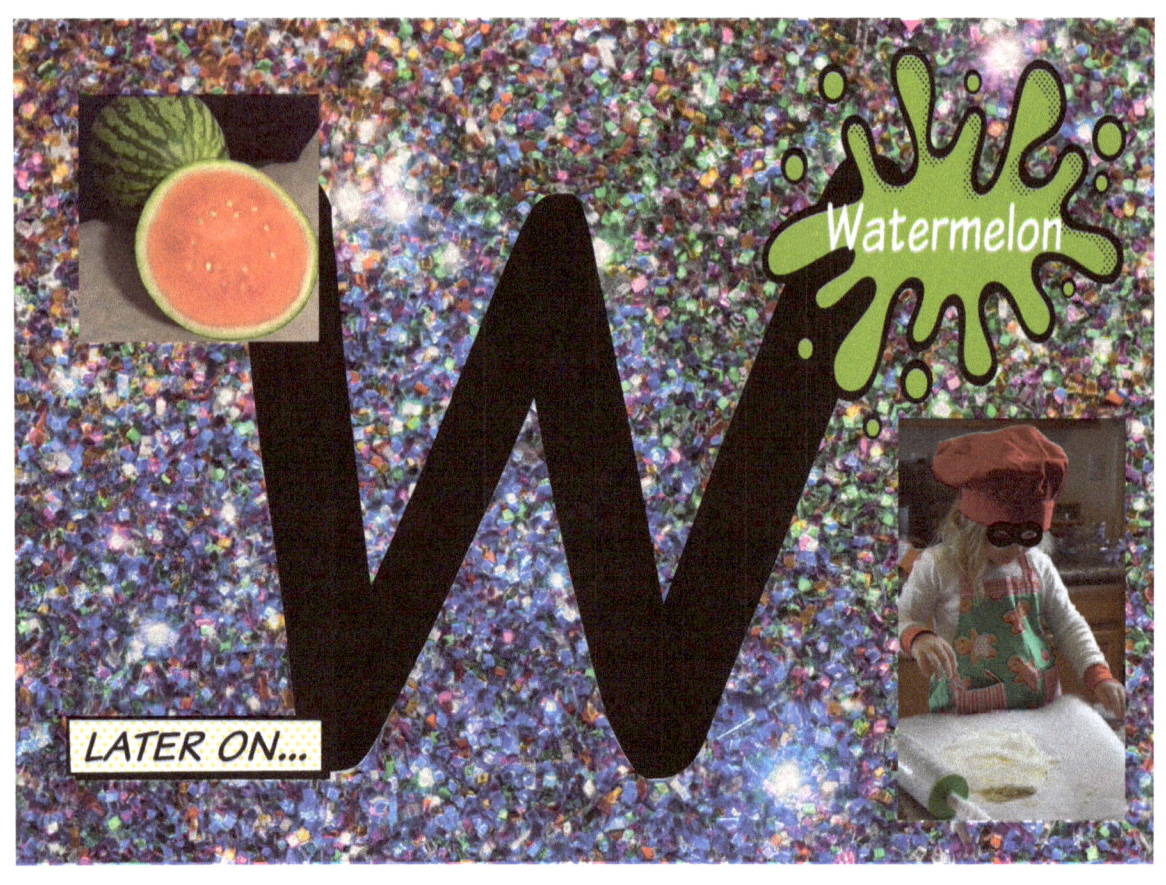

Watermelon is sweet and juicy originating in West Africa.

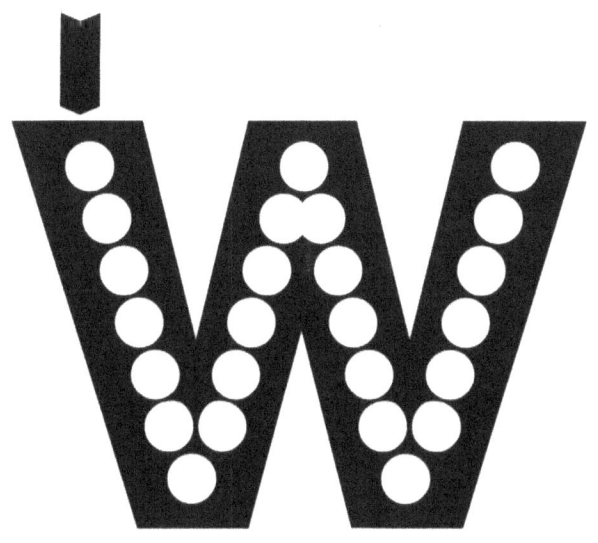

W is for Water.

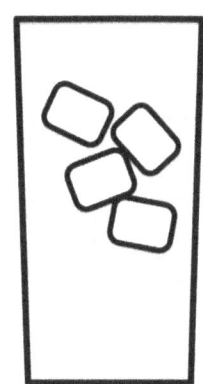

WE NEED TO DRINK WATER TO LIVE.

Ww

Practice writing the letter W.

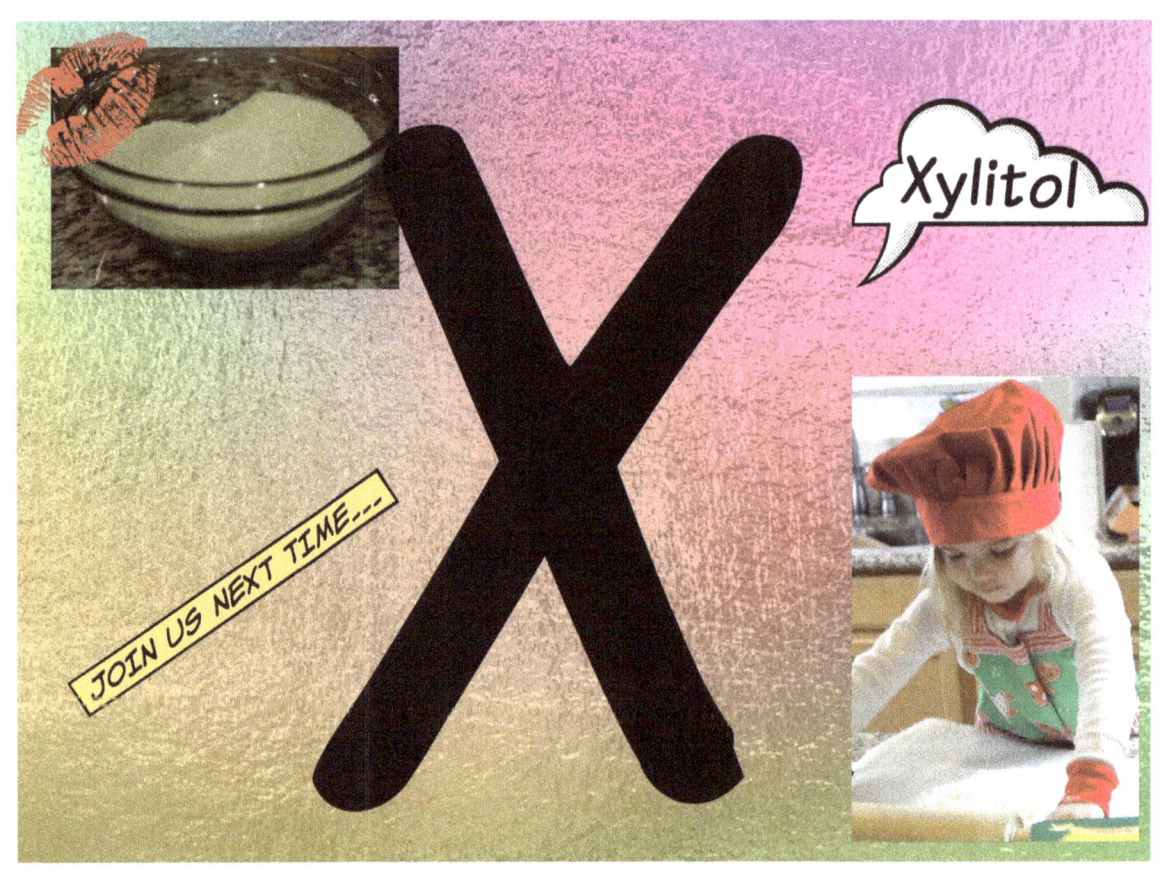

Xylitol is a sugar alcohol and is found to prevent ear infections.

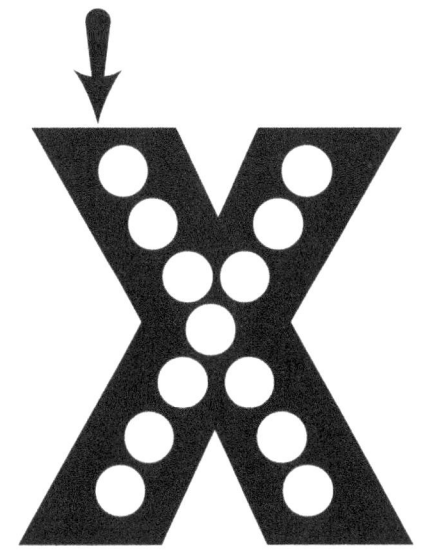

X is for Xylitol.

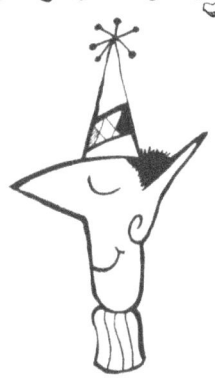

XYLITOL HELPS PREVENT EAR INFECTIONS AND IS A SWEETNER, TOO.

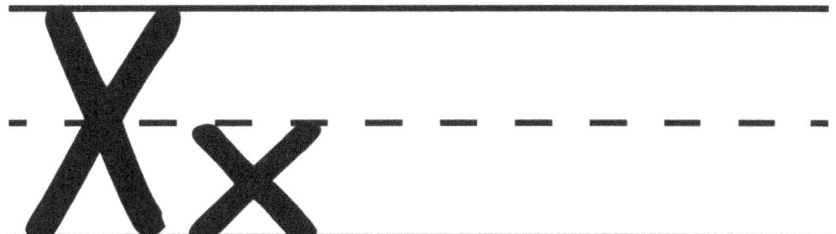

Practice writing the letter X.

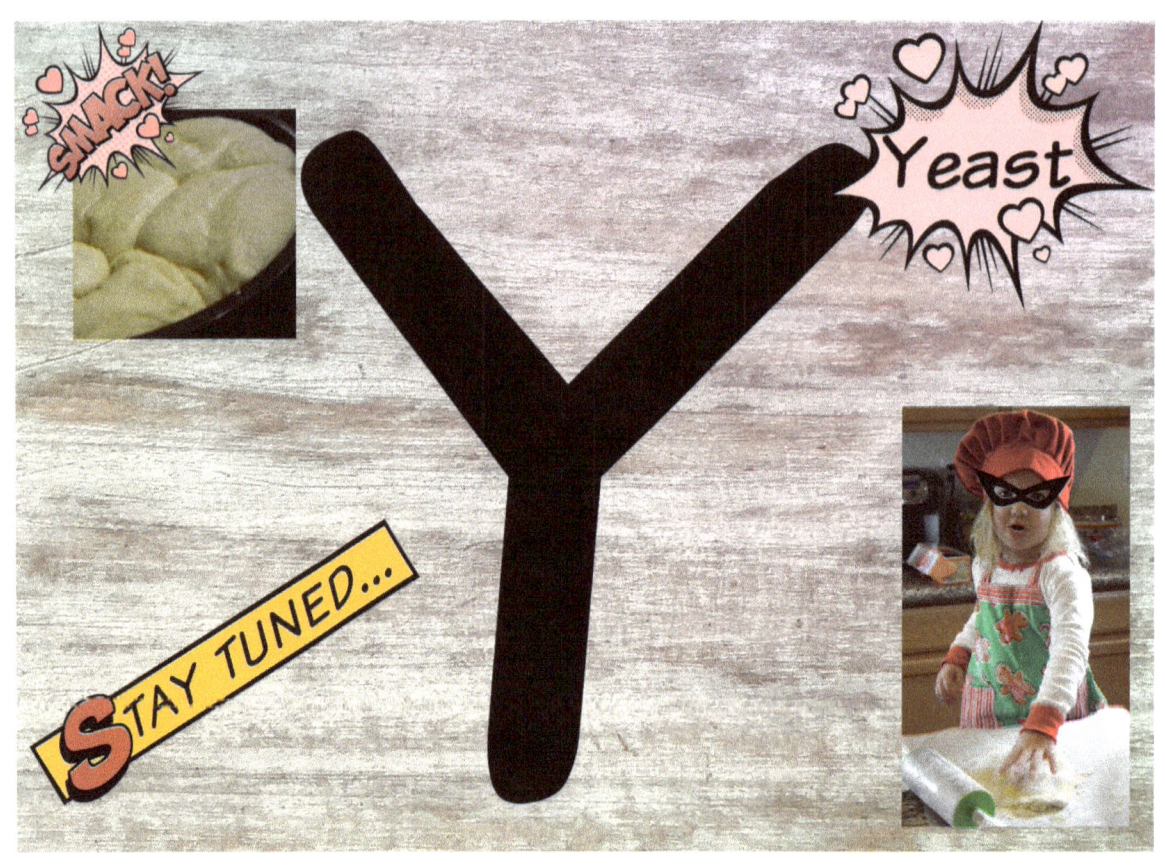

Yeast makes dough rise and baked goods fluffy.

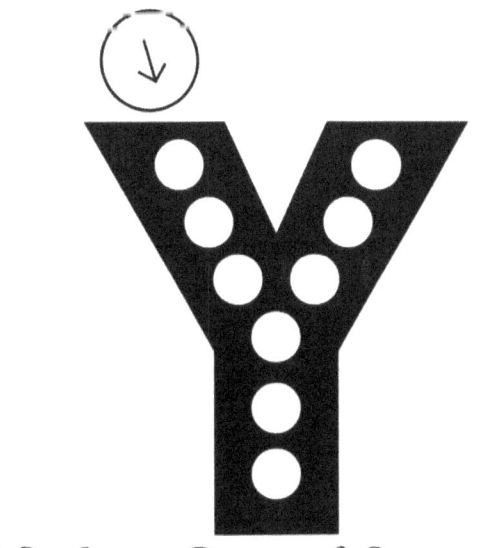

Y is for Yeast.

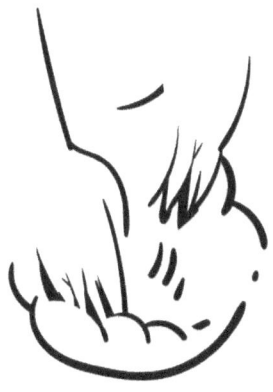

YEAST MAKES BREAD RISE SO IT IS SOFT AND GOOD.

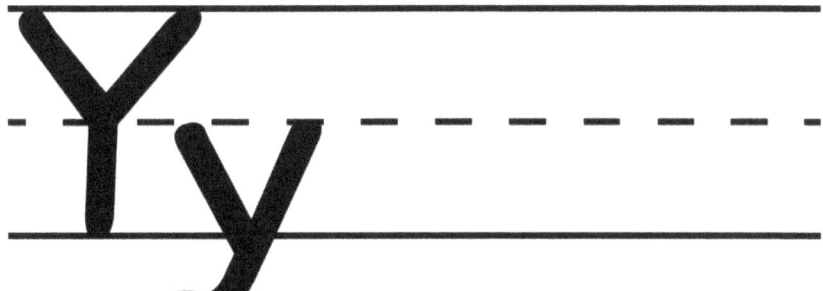

Practice writing the letter Y.

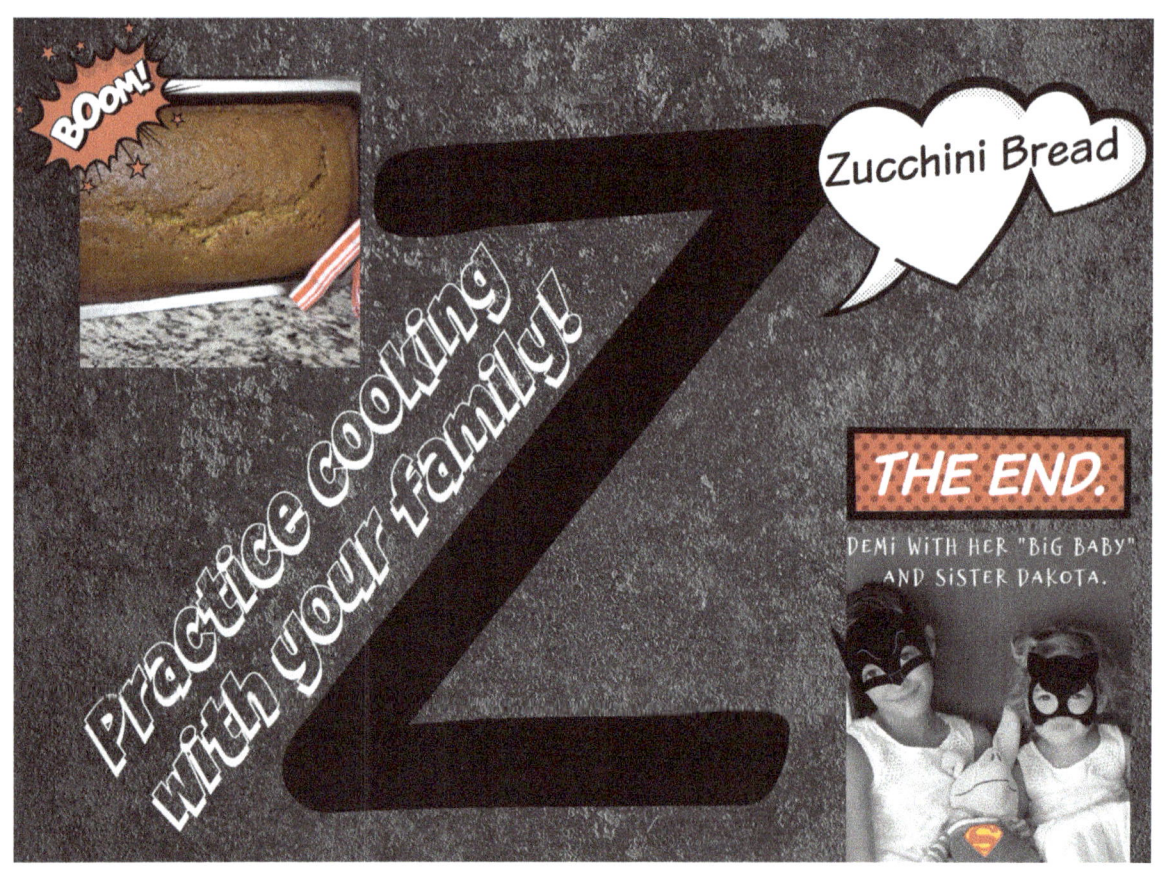

Zucchini is a vegetable that can be used when making bread.

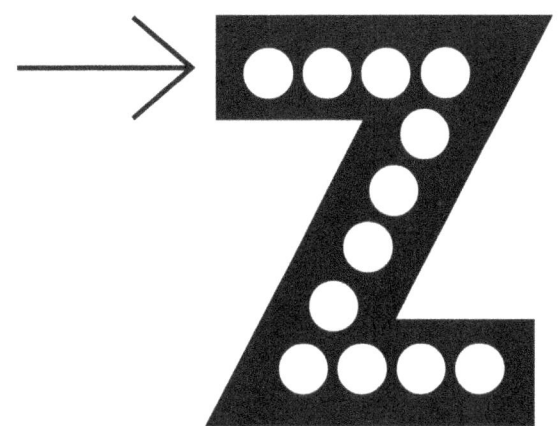

Z is for Zucchini.

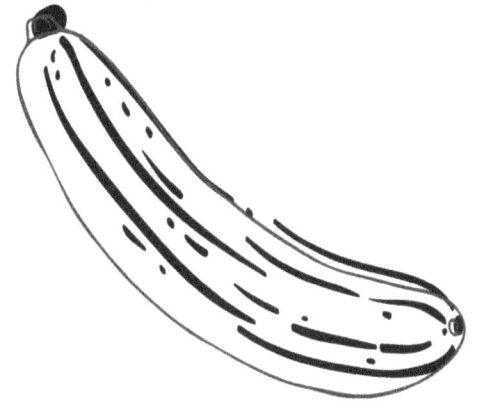

ZUCCHINI OR BANANA CAN BE USED IN BREAD.

Zz

Practice writing the letter Z.

Name _____

WRITE LETTERS
_____

Practice writing your letters.

Name _____

WRITE LETTERS

Practice writing your letters.

Name _____

WRITE LETTERS

Aa

Aa

Aa

Aa

Aa

Practice writing the letter A.

Name _____

WRITE LETTERS

Bb ---------------

Bb ---------------

Bb ---------------

Bb ---------------

Bb ---------------

Practice writing the letter B.

Name _____

WRITE LETTERS

Cc *Cc* ----------------

Cc *Cc* ----------------

Cc *Cc* ----------------

Cc *Cc* ----------------

Cc *Cc* ----------------

Practice writing the letter C.

Name _____

WRITE LETTERS

Dd
Dd
Dd
Dd
Dd

Practice writing the letter D.

Name _____

WRITE LETTERS

Ee — — — — — — — — — — —

Ee — — — — — — — — — — —

Ee — — — — — — — — — — —

Ee — — — — — — — — — — —

Ee — — — — — — — — — — —

Practice writing the letter E.

Name _____

WRITE LETTERS

Ff — — — — — — — — — — —

Ff — — — — — — — — — — —

Ff — — — — — — — — — — —

Ff — — — — — — — — — — —

Ff — — — — — — — — — — —

Practice writing the letter F.

Name _____

WRITE LETTERS

Gg ----

Gg ----

Gg ----

Gg ----

Gg ----

Practice writing
the letter G.

Name _____

WRITE LETTERS

Hh — — — — — — —

Hh — — — — — — —

Hh — — — — — — —

Hh — — — — — — —

Hh — — — — — — —

Practice writing the letter H.

Name _____

WRITE LETTERS

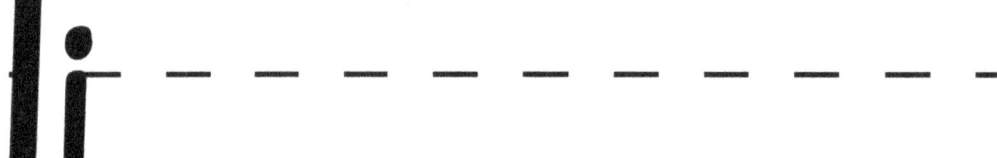

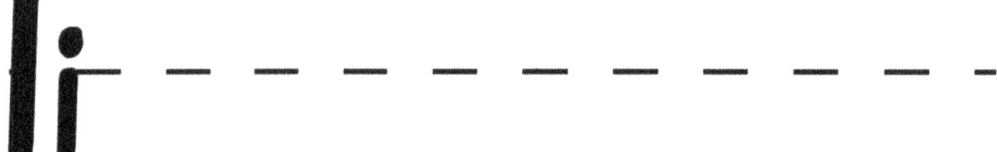

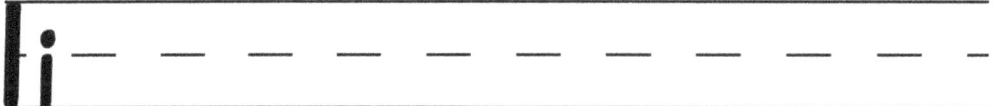

Practice writing the letter I.

Name _____

WRITE LETTERS

Jj

Jj

Jj

Jj

Jj

Practice writing
the letter J.

Name _____

WRITE LETTERS

Kk --------
Kk --------
Kk --------
Kk --------
Kk --------

Practice writing the letter K.

Name _____

WRITE LETTERS

Ll

Ll

Ll

Ll

Ll

Practice writing the letter L.

Name _____

WRITE LETTERS

Mm -----------

Mm -----------

Mm -----------

Mm -----------

Mm -----------

Practice writing the letter M.

Name _____

WRITE LETTERS

Nn
Nn
Nn
Nn
Nn

Practice writing
the letter N.

Name _____

WRITE LETTERS

Oo -- -- -- -- -- -- -- --

Oo -- -- -- -- -- -- -- --

Oo -- -- -- -- -- -- -- --

Oo -- -- -- -- -- -- -- --

Oo -- -- -- -- -- -- -- --

Practice writing the letter O.

Name _____

WRITE LETTERS

Pp

Pp

Pp

Pp

Pp

Practice writing the letter P.

Name _____

WRITE LETTERS

Qq

Qq

Qq

Qq

Qq

Practice writing
the letter Q.

Name _____

WRITE LETTERS

Rr -------------------

Rr -------------------

Rr -------------------

Rr -------------------

Rr -------------------

Practice writing
the letter R.

Name _____

WRITE LETTERS

Ss -----------------

Ss -----------------

Ss -----------------

Ss -----------------

Ss -----------------

Practice writing the letter S.

Name _____

WRITE LETTERS

Tt

Tt

Tt

Tt

Tt

Practice writing the letter T.

Name _____

WRITE LETTERS

Uu — — — — — — — —

Uu — — — — — — — —

Uu — — — — — — — —

Uu — — — — — — — —

Uu — — — — — — — —

Practice writing the letter U.

Name _____

WRITE LETTERS

Vv

Vv

Vv

Vv

Vv

Practice writing the letter V.

Name _____

WRITE LETTERS

Ww ---------------

Ww ---------------

Ww ---------------

Ww ---------------

Ww ---------------

Practice writing
the letter W.

Name _____

WRITE LETTERS

Xx
Xx
Xx
Xx
Xx

Practice writing the letter X.

Name _____

WRITE LETTERS

Yy

Yy

Yy

Yy

Yy

Practice writing the letter Y.

Name _____

WRITE LETTERS

Zz

Zz

Zz

Zz

Zz

Practice writing the letter Z.

Name _____

WRITE LETTERS

Practice writing your letters.

www.ingramcontent.com/pod-product-compliance
Lightning Source LLC
Chambersburg PA
CBHW061151070526
44584CB00034B/4478